A LITTLE NIP, A LITTLE TUCK

An Insiders Guide to Cosmetic Enhancement

By Stephen T. Greenberg, MD, FACS

Board Certified Aesthetic Plastic Surgeon

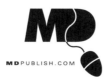

MDPUBLISH.COM

ISBN-13: 978-0-9748997-7-0   ISBN-13: 978-0-9792240-1-0
ISBN-10: 0-9748997-7-1   ISBN-10: 0-9792240-1-2
(Softcover)   (Hardcover)

Printed in the United States of America.

Cover concept and design by The Egc Group
Book design by StarGraphics Studio

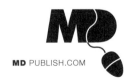

MD PUBLISH.COM   350 Fifth Avenue, Suite 7619 | New York, New York 10118

About Dr. Greenberg

Stephen T. Greenberg, MD is a nationally recognized aesthetic plastic surgeon. He received his medical degree with highest distinction from George Washington University. He then completed his surgical training at the prestigious New York Hospital-Cornell University Medical Center. He subsequently trained in Plastic and Reconstructive surgery at the Hospital of the University of Pennsylvania. He is board certified by both the American Board of Plastic Surgery and the American Board of Surgery. Dr. Greenberg is an active member of the American Society of Plastic Surgeons, and an active member of the New York Regional Society of Plastic Surgeons, The Nassau County Medical Society, and the American Medical Association.

Dr. Greenberg is the medical director of one of the most advanced cosmetic surgical centers, with locations in Woodbury, Long Island, and New York City where he offers the full range of cosmetic surgical procedures for women and men. Dr. Greenberg's team is comprised of aestheticians, nurses, makeup artists, hair stylists, and a nutritionist, cosmetic dentist, and fitness trainer.

Dr. Greenberg is frequently sought after by the media for his expertise in plastic surgery. He has been featured on the *CBS Evening News with Dan Rather*, on *Inside Edition*, NBC, CBS, and *Good Morning America*. In addition, Dr. Greenberg has been featured on the front covers of both the *New York Times* and Newsday, has been interviewed by a host of women's magazines including *Cosmopolitan*, *Harper's Bazaar*, *Elle*, and many others. Dr. Greenberg hosts his own cosmetic surgery radio talk shows on WKJY, 98.3 FM and on 105.3 FM and 107.1 FM in New York.

Stephen T. Greenberg, MD, F.A.C.S., PC
Board-Certified Plastic Surgeon
461 Park Avenue South
New York, NY 10021
212-319-4999
195 Froehlich Farm Blvd
Woodbury, NY 11797
516-364-4200
www.greenbergcosmeticsurgery.com

Acknowledgments

I would like to thank Lisa Kaufman, my staff, nurses, and anesthesiologists for their exceptional commitment to patient care. To the team at MDPUBLISH, thank you for making this book a reality for me.

Dedication

To my children and family, with extreme gratitude for their support and encouragement during the writing of this book. I would also like to thank my parents for their support, encouragement and love. To my wonderful staff who work tirelessly, and to my many patients who generously share their experience with others and who make all this possible.

Contents

THE FACE

FINISHING TOUCHES

Introduction

Wallis Simpson, the Duchess of Windsor, once said, "You can never be too rich or too thin." Most of us feel that you can never be too beautiful for a little nip and tuck. At some point, every one of us secretly wishes for a little work, and there's no shame in that!

Our youth oriented culture accepts the idea of improving one's image. In fact, some might say, we embrace it with open arms. My practice draws chic Manhattanites, busy urban professionals, and suburban housewives seeking an image boost. Our clients run the gamut from teens in search of thinner thighs to their moms who are seeking the fountain of youth, to celebrities and supermodels. I have seen my share of drama in the operating room: demanding divas, sexy socialites, frenzied fashionistas, and the rest of us who want to look like them.

My office is a constant bustle of energy, which has a lot to do with the many improvements in cosmetic surgery procedures in the last few years. Advancements in technology and methods that make procedures safer and more effective with less recovery have made plastic surgery increasingly popular. Safety has become a major concern for patients. Everyone has read the horror stories about botched Botox® and unscrupulous doctors operating without a license. While these are isolated cases, patients have become savvy consumers, and they are doing their homework, whether they are going in for a syringe of Restylane® or for a mini-facelift. The truth is, cosmetic surgery is very safe as long as it is done correctly by a qualified plastic surgeon. This means educating yourself about what you want, what is possible, and what is just a figment of reality television's collective imagination. If you feel comfortable with the first doctor you see, he or she may be the right fit for you.

The extreme makeover concept opened doors for women and men who never imagined they could be beautiful and desirable. The trend is no longer confined to adults alone. As a new generation of fabulous starlets is getting younger and thinner—and more and more beautiful with every magazine snapshot—young women aren't just buying the clothes that their favorite celebrities are wearing. They want to become the next Lindsay Lohan or Jessica Simpson. What was once considered unattainable is now within the reach of many. It seems completely realistic these days to walk into your doctor's office and walk out with the breasts or nose that you should have been born with. This book will show you step-by-step how you can go from glum to glam.

There's no doubt that plastic surgery has been given a lot of press coverage in the last year. According to the American Society of Plastic Surgeons, this year's Hot Topics in Plastic Surgery include:

- **Only the rich and famous; think again**—In an age when beauty is gender-blind, men are turning to cosmetic surgery *en masse*, without the fear and stigma that once accompanied it. The simple fact is that cosmetic surgery is going where no procedure has gone before to restore youth and beauty. Looking as good as you can is no longer just for the wealthy. A study brought by the ASPS reports that most people who are contemplating cosmetic surgery have a combined household income of less than $60,000. Those who make over $90,000 account for only 13 percent of candidates.

- **No endorsement for mesotherapy**—A recent study shows there is no evidence proving the safety and long-term efficacy of mesotherapy. None of the substances used to inject patients is approved by the FDA, and there is no standardization of technique.

- **Injectables fill the market**—Less invasive forms of image enhancement are also on the rise. Gone are the days when you had to schedule an appointment months in advance to smooth out wrinkles or add volume to your face. My patients come to me for a touch up every six months or so, and they walk out looking much younger. Cosmetic patients have more minimally invasive options today with the advent of injectable wrinkle fillers and laser technologies. ASPS reported that minimally invasive procedures climbed 36 percent.

- **Diversity among plastic surgery patients**—More than 1.3 million cosmetic plastic surgery procedures were performed on ethnic patients in 2004, an increase of 44 percent since 2000. Fourteen percent of all cosmetic plastic surgery patients were Asian, Black, or Hispanic. These patients have similar motivations as other patients, and often prefer to maintain their ethnic identity while achieving a more youthful appearance.

- **No new taxes**—In a subtle but important victory for the average American, lawmakers in several states elected not to impose a tax on cosmetic procedures. Legislation was considered in Illinois, Washington, New York, Tennessee, Texas, and Arkansas when budgets came up short.

- **Silicone breast implants are back**—Breast augmentation is among the most popular cosmetic procedures. In 2005, after 13 years of restricted access, the Food and Drug Administration (FDA) deemed silicone implants from manufacturers Allergan and Mentor approvable with conditions. In the fall of 2006, the ban was repealed and silicone breast implants returned to the market for breast reconstruction and cosmetic breast augmentation, with limited cosmetic use in women 22 and older.

- **Manufacturers investing in the future**—Looking to boost their position in the fast-growing cosmetic plastic surgery market, several large plastic surgery product companies have begun efforts to acquire other manufacturers. Focused around breast implants and injectable wrinkle fighters, these companies hope to capitalize on the highly demanding baby boomers.

Unfortunately, the obesity epidemic in the United States is on the rise. Cosmetic surgery is literally picking up the slack with body contouring. People who lose a few dress sizes often have a new battle to fight—slack, hanging skin that just will not budge with diet and exercise. Bodylifts can remove excess skin from the breasts, arms, tummy, hips, and thighs.

This is an exciting time in plastic surgery. Innovations in technology and techniques lead the way while a more diverse range of patients seek procedures. The time to change your life and look like one in a million is now. The only thing stopping you from taking that next step is YOU.

CHAPTER 1

Choosing Doctor Right

An Investment for Life

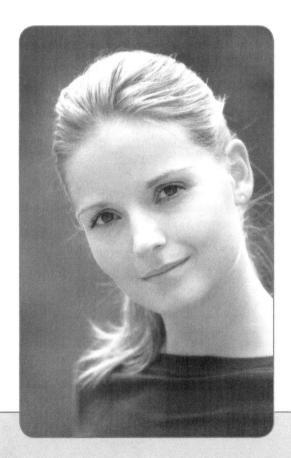

C osmetic surgery is booming—and why not? The procedures are safe and the results can be amazing. You are about to invest in a purchase whose outcome will affect the rest of your life. Finding the best plastic surgeon for your procedure is the most important step in your journey. Get ready for some serious attention, because with my help, no one will be able to take their eyes off the sexy new you!

Greenberg's Myths about Plastic Surgery Dispelled

Botox® is poison

Everyone who gets a facelift looks fake like Joan Rivers

After eyelid surgery, you won't be able to close your eyes when you go to sleep

You can always spot fake breasts

When you have liposuction, the fat is going to go somewhere else

If you have a browlift, you will always look surprised

What's Hot
- Credentials matter, so only go with a doctor who is certified by the American Board of Plastic Surgery
- Independent surgery centers certified by The American Association for Accreditation of Ambulatory Surgery Facilities (AAAASF)
- Enhancing your looks, your outlook, and your self-confidence safely with plastic surgery
- Getting tons of reliable, objective information to help you make the best decision when it comes to your appearance
- Natural results are the only way to go

What's Not
- Doctors who are not plastic surgeons, performing cosmetic surgical procedures
- Unrealistic expectations or promises
- Fake-looking results
- Long recoveries
- Ugly, visible scars

From the minute you step into the initial consultation, you should feel like all eyes are on you. Your surgeon should be attentive and patient. You should feel comfortable with both the doctor and the office staff, and you have the right to have all your questions answered. Many individuals prefer to go on a few consultations before settling on a doctor. However, if you like the doctor and get the answers you need to the questions below, one may do the trick.

FAST FACTS ABOUT COSMETIC SURGERY (ASAPS 2005)

Women make up 91.4 percent of cosmetic surgery patients in the U.S.

Americans age 35-50 have the largest number of procedures.

Almost 48 percent of procedures are performed in office-based facilities.

Top five surgical procedures are: liposuction, breast augmentation, eyelid surgery, rhinoplasty and abdominoplasty.

Top five non-surgical procedures are: Botox®, laser hair removal, hyaluronic acids, microdermabrasion, and chemical peels.

Most common procedures after massive weight loss are liposuction, tummy tucks, lower bodylifts, upper armlifts, and thighlifts.

From Consumer Survey of 1000 American Households (ASAPS 2006)

Americans' general approval of cosmetic surgery:

- 55 percent of women say they approve of cosmetic surgery
- 52 percent of men say they approve of cosmetic surgery

Would consider cosmetic surgery for self, now or in the future:

- 32 percent of women
- 19 percent of men

Would not be embarrassed about having cosmetic surgery:

- 82 percent of women say that, if they had cosmetic surgery in the future, they would not be embarrassed if people outside their immediate family and close friends knew about it

- 79 percent of men would not be embarrassed

Would consider cosmetic surgery for self, now or in the future, by age [includes both men and women]:

- 14 percent of Americans age 65 or older
- 27 percent of 55-64 year olds
- 23 percent of 45-54 year olds
- 29 percent of 35-44 year olds
- 30 percent of 25-34 year olds
- 30 percent of 18-24 year olds

Would consider cosmetic surgery for self, now or in the future, by marital status [includes both men and women]:

- 25 percent of married Americans
- 28 percent of unmarried Americans

Would consider cosmetic surgery for self, now or in the future by race/ethnicity [includes both men and women]:

- 26 percent of white Americans
- 25 percent of non-white Americans

Would consider cosmetic surgery for self, now or in the future by child in household [includes both men and women]:

- 30 percent of Americans with child in household
- 23 percent of Americans with no child in household

Finding the right surgeon is about looking for the right match to make you feel confident.

Be prepared to take this handy checklist with you to the consultation.

Tips for Kicking Off Your Search for a Surgeon

HAPPY PATIENTS Happy Patients: Nothing beats a referral from a satisfied patient. If you admire your best friend's nose job or your neighbor's facelift or breasts, you will have a better idea of what you can expect from their doctor.

A DOCTOR YOU TRUST Ask your gynecologist, pediatrician, family doctor, or any other MD you trust for a recommendation. You would be surprised at how small the medical community is, and doctors know other docs both personally and by reputation. Verify the physician's medical certifications, membership in professional societies, and medical license.

Be sure to check out the surgeon's personal website to get the full flavor of his or her practice.

SURFING THE NET FOR YOUR MD
Dr. Greenberg's Top 5 Websites

www.platicsurgery.org The American Society of Plastic Surgeons

www.surgery.org The American Society for Aesthetic Plastic Surgery

www.abps.org American Board of Plastic Surgery

www.abms.org American Board of Medical Specialties

www.mentorcorp.org Mentor Corp

Radio and Television Listening to a doctor on the radio or television can be a helpful jumping off point to start your research, but make sure that you ask all the following questions to ensure the doctor is right for you.

Price Whether you are on a tight budget or are living the life of a socialite, money should never be the deciding factor when it comes to your health and your appearance. It is not the only measure of value or quality, so don't make your decision based on price. The most expensive surgeon is not necessarily the best. At the same time, there is no such thing as a discount on quality and skilled care.

GREENBERG'S LIST
Top Questions for Your Consultation

Before you hop on the operating room table, you'll need to consider a few things. Some of these questions can be answered by the receptionist when you schedule your appointment. Others can be found on the doctor's website. Some you should ask the doctor directly. Remember, even if you know the answers to some of these questions, it never hurts to ask. You need to know whether the surgeon is being upfront, downplaying the risks, or exaggerating the benefits.

Don't be afraid to ask a lot of questions. Probe further to get a straight answer if the responses to your queries are evasive or incomplete.

Is the doctor board-certified and, if so, by whom?

> *The only acceptable answer is: "YES! The doctor is board-certified by The American Board of Plastic Surgery."*

The American Board of Plastic Surgery is the only board exclusive to plastic surgery. Physicians holding ABPS certification are the only ones certified to perform all types of plastic surgery, of the face and body. You can confirm certification directly through the American Board of Plastic Surgery (www.abps.org). By choosing a board-certified plastic surgeon, you know the doctor has graduated from an accredited medical school and has completed at least five years of additional training as a resident surgeon (a minimum of three years in an accredited general surgery program and two years in plastic surgery). To become certified, the doctor must then successfully complete comprehensive written and oral exams. Board certification is a voluntary process. The mission of the American Board of Plastic Surgery is to promote safe, ethical plastic surgery to the public by maintaining high standards for the education, examination, certification, and re-certification of plastic surgery specialties.

Check the surgeon's medical education and training in cosmetic surgery. Confirm the number of similar procedures done by the physician and how often such surgeries are performed. Since surgeons are not experts in all areas, a surgeon who did a good facelift for your friend might not be suitable for doing a breast augmentation. Go through "before and after" photographs of patients who have undergone surgery and assess the results.

> The American Society of Plastic Surgeons and the American Society for Aesthetic Plastic Surgery have rigorous standards for training requirements and enforcing ethical practices. Other societies may simply be a professional association. Many are just clubs or groups that have limited requirements to become members.

Being a licensed medical doctor is not enough, since doctors don't get their license in one specialty. This means the doctor can provide any medical service he or she desires. Any doctor can legally offer plastic surgery or cosmetic services of any kind, regardless of his or her education, board certification (or lack thereof), training, or skill level.

> *As scary as it may sound, this means that an internist, pediatrician, or psychiatrist can insert breast implants or inject Botox®.*

MEDICAL SOCIETIES THAT MAKE THE CUT

The American Society of Plastic Surgeons (ASPS)
www.plasticsurgery.org
Founded in 1931, the ASPS is the largest plastic and reconstructive surgery specialty organization in the world. Members of ASPS are required to operate only in accredited or licensed surgical facilities.

CONTINUED

The American Society for Aesthetic Plastic Surgery (ASAPS)
www.surgery.org

Since 1967, ASAPS has been among the leading organizations for aesthetic plastic surgery education and research. Members have met specific requirements for clinical experience, ethics, and continuing education in cosmetic surgery. They are required to operate only in accredited or licensed surgical facilities and must complete a stated number of continuing medical education hours specific to patient safety.

The American Academy of Facial Plastic and Reconstructive Surgeons (AAFPRS)
www.aafrs.org

Since 1964, the AAFPRS represents facial plastic and reconstructive surgeons certified by the American Board of Otolaryngology to perform plastic and reconstructive procedures of the face, head, and neck only.

The American Society for Dermatologic Surgery (ASDS)
www.asds-net.org

Members of the ASDS, founded in 1970, are board-certified dermatologists with additional accredited continuing medical education and research of procedures to maintain the health, function, and aesthetic appearance of the skin, hair, and nails.

The American Academy of Dermatology (AAD)
www.aad.org

Members of AAD are board-certified dermatologists specializing in the medical and cosmetic treatment of the skin, hair, and nails.

The American Society of Ophthalmic Plastic and Reconstructive Surgery (ASOPRS)
www.asoprs.org

The ASOPRS was founded in 1969 and is exclusive to board-certified ophthalmologists. ASOPRS focused on the training, education, research, and quality of clinical practice in cosmetic and reconstructive surgery of the eyelids and orbital region.

Where does the doctor perform surgery?

Many years ago outpatient procedures were limited. With modern technology, doctors can do many more surgeries outside the hospital, and they have a lot more leeway with the types of medication and anesthesia they can use. Thankfully, the patient also has less post-operative pain and usually doesn't have to stay in bed after the procedure. Techniques, technology, and even the general approach to cosmetic surgery have changed. However, just because plastic surgery is safer, easier, and less painful, it is still major surgery. We haven't minimized the type of surgery; we've just maximized the efficiency and the results.

Any independent ambulatory surgery center must be accredited by the American Association of Ambulatory Surgery Facilities or AAAASF (www.aaasf.org). If the center is not accredited, RUN! For safety's sake, the surgeon must have privileges to perform your procedure in a hospital. This shows that the plastic surgeon's credentials have been reviewed and meet the hospital's standards.

A fully-accredited facility has more flexibility than a hospital when it comes to scheduling your surgery; it provides a cohesive, familiar team of doctors, nurses, and anesthesiologists who work together daily; and there is a more private, calmer environment, which has the added benefit of being more cost-effective. However, if you are having multiple procedures or have prior medical problems, it may make sense to have your procedures performed in a hospital.

Documentation of accreditation may also come from one of these governing bodies: Accreditation Association for Ambulatory Health Care (AAAHC) and Joint Commission on Accreditation of Healthcare Organizations (JCAHO). Regulations for freestanding clinics and surgicenters fall under federal as well as state and local standards.

How long has the doctor been in practice?

There is no right or wrong answer to this question, but five years is a good place to start. It is a matter of your comfort level. Experience counts.

Does the doctor have any specialties or favorite procedures?

Sometimes surgeons become known as "face doctors" or "breast doctors." Find out which procedures the surgeon performs most frequently and why.

Who will be assisting the doctor in the operating room?

Generally, you can expect one anesthesiologist, one operating room technician, and one registered nurse in an independent surgery center.

Who are the anesthesiologists and how long have they been working with the doctor? Do they also work in hospitals?

Obviously, the longer the doctor has worked with the anesthesiologist, the better. It's also optimal if the anesthesiologist works in a hospital as well. Make sure the doctor clearly defines the anesthesia you will have and the credentials of the person who will administer it. For the most part, anesthesia will be administered by an anesthesiologist, (an M.D. who has completed an accredited residency in anesthesiology). For limited procedures that are performed with topical or local anesthetic and oral sedation alone, your surgeon may administer the anesthesia.

ALL ABOUT ANESTHESIA
What to Expect?

Local (topical or injectable) A topical cream is applied to the treatment site in advance, or an injection at the treatment site will numb only that area.

Local with Sedation A "conscious sedation" involves a local anesthetic administered topically or by injection; a nerve block via injection; or sedation drugs (like Valium) administered through an IV or orally. IV sedation should be performed only by an appropriate anesthesia provider in an accredited or licensed facility in order to adequately monitor the patient and assure safety.

Regional An epidural used during childbirth is a perfect example of regional anesthesia. This type of anesthetic eliminates pain in a larger area of the body via an injection. It blocks a group of nerves so the pain cannot reach the brain.

General Usually involves inhaling an anesthesia gas, which puts the patient to sleep and prevents any feeling of pain. General anesthetic can be used with or without controlled breathing through a tube in the throat. General anesthesia should be performed only in an accredited or licensed facility in order to adequately monitor the patient and assure safety, and only under the direction of a trained anesthesia provider, such as an anesthesiologist or certified registered nurse anesthetist.

PRE-ANESTHESIA QUESTIONS

Is there is any chance you could be pregnant, or are you nursing?

What was the date of your last menstrual period?

What medications are you currently taking?

Have you or any family member had any problems with anesthesia?

Do you have any allergies to medications?

Are you a smoker?

When was the last time you ate or drank?

Do you bruise easily or have excessive bleeding from tooth extractions and menstrual cycles?

What types of incisions/scarring can you expect?

The plastic surgeon's job is to make you look better. For some procedures, scars are unavoidable but for many procedures, scars should be minimal or not even visible. If you have a history of bad scarring or thickened scars such as keloids, you should inform your physician ahead of time. In general, the immediate scars will remain somewhat thickened for weeks and often months, then gradually become less obvious, ideally eventually fading to thin lines.

It takes about one year for scars to fully fade. Scarring is unpredictable and depends on the patients' own genetics and many other factors. The surgeon can never promise how your scar is going to heal.

How long is the procedure?

PROCEDURE	AVERAGE TIME
Facelift with Eyelids	4-6 Hours
Upper or Lower Eyelids	45 Minutes
Upper and Lower Eyelids	1-1 ½ Hours
Browlift	1 Hour
Facelift	2-3 Hours
Rhinoplasty	1-2 Hours
Breast Augmentation	1 Hour
Breastlift or Reduction	2-3 Hours
Liposuction	1-2 Hours
Tummy Tuck	2 Hours
Bodylift	3 Hours
Armlift	2-4 Hours

What can you expect after surgery?

Listen carefully to the doctor when the recovery period is discussed. This is a practical issue that will help you to plan your surgery during a time that allows full recovery and takes into account work and family issues. Everyone heals differently.

COSMETIC SURGERY RECOVER TIMES
A General Guideline

Back home Same day or next day

Shower 1-2 days

Washing your hair 1-2 days

Dressing removal Next day

Suture removal 3-7 days

Staple removal 4-10 days

Surgical drain removal 1-7 days

Aerobic exercise 3-4 weeks

Bruising up to 3 weeks

Makeup 7-10 days

How long is the recovery?

The real deal on recovery is the earliest possible date when you can put on concealing makeup, fix your hair, and go back to work comfortably, looking and feeling "semi-normal."

BACK TO WORK

Upper eyelid lifts 5-7 days

Lower eyelid fat bag removal 5-7 days

Facelift 10 - 14 days

Liposuction 2-4 days

Tummy Tuck 2 weeks

Bodylift 2-3 weeks

Breast Augmentation 2 days

Breastlift/Reduction 3 days

What is the complication rate and touch up rate?

Although cosmetic surgery is safer than ever, there's not a doctor in the world who has never had a complication or an unhappy patient. The odds are against it. Listen for honest answers.

Can you speak to previous patients?

It's wonderful and reassuring to speak with at least one of the surgeon's patients who had the same procedure you are considering.

Do you have before/after photographs?

Again, for your peace of mind, I highly recommend that you look at the surgeon's photographs. If he or she does not have photographs of your procedure, you can safely assume it is not their specialty. The idea is to choose a surgeon who is known for the work you are looking to have done.

How long will results last?

This depends on other factors including genetics, lifestyle, whether you smoke or drink, and the type of surgery you have had.

PROCEDURE	HOW LONG IT SHOULD LAST
Facelift with Eyelids	5-10 years
Upper and Lower Eyelids	5-10 years
Browlift	5-10 years
Rhinoplasty	Permanent
Breast Augmentation	15 years—variable, can be permanent
Breastlift or Reduction	10 years—variable, can be permanent
Liposuction	Permanent if you keep your weight stable
Bodylift	10 years, can be permanent if no weight surges
Tummy Tuck	10 years, can be permanent if no weight surges
Armlift	10 years, can be permanent if no weight surges

Is there a fee for follow up visits?

Most surgeons do not charge another fee for follow up visits after you have had surgery. This should be discussed beforehand.

How many follow up visits will there be?

This will vary depending on how close you live to the surgeon and the type of procedure you are having done. For example, after a facelift, most patients will need to be seen two to three times for suture and dressing removal in the first two weeks. The next follow up visit may be scheduled at six weeks, 12 weeks, six months, and one year. If there are any complications, you may need to be seen more often.

How many of these procedures does the doctor do each month?

Five should be the minimum; or at least one per week.

What are the risks?

It is your right to know about the potential risks and complications before surgery. Although your doctor should make every effort to minimize complications, it is not possible to eliminate the potential for all problems from occurring. With any surgical procedure, there is always a possibility of unexpected or unwanted events. No absolute guarantees as to the final result can ever be given by any physician.

The risks of cosmetic surgery can be divided into two main groups: those that are common after all operations, and those that are unique to a specific technique or procedure. It is also important to factor in the variables of your individual health status, your age, skin quality, gender, and your medical history. A younger patient in prime health will have less risks than an older patient with a history of high blood pressure. Males are more prone to bleeding because they have a rich blood supply and thicker skin. Thin skinned patients may be more prone to bruising.

The most common risks of cosmetic procedures include swelling, bruising, bleeding, infection, prolonged numbness, and a reaction to anesthesia. General surgical complications may include hematoma, which is a blood clot; seroma which is a collection of clear fluid; nerve damage, scar tissue formation, asymmetries, and irregularities. Infections are rare and are typically treated with a course of antibiotics. It is common to have an antibiotic prescribed before and/or after surgery to guard against infection. If you are having a surgery that involves placing an implant or graft, there is always the possibility of extrusion, whereby the implant works its way up to the surface of the skin; and capsular contracture, which is an excess tightening of scar tissue that forms around the implant.

Smoking can increase the risks of this procedure because nicotine constricts the blood vessels, decreases blood flow to tissues, and greatly increases the chance of scarring. In some cases, smokers can actually lose a portion of skin due to decreased oxygen flow into the skin caused by carbon monoxide. All forms, including nicotine substitutes and smoker's aids, can increase the risk of poor healing, skin sloughing, scabbing and crusting. These risks are significantly reduced if you stop smoking at least two weeks before surgery and wait until you are completely healed before starting again, or preferably, quit smoking entirely. However, even if you exercise these precautions, there are no guarantees.

After the procedure, you will be instructed to be on the lookout for the signs of infection near the incisions: increased swelling, redness, high fever, warmth, bleeding, or other discharge. If you experience any unusual symptoms, such as heavy bleeding, throbbing, or sudden pain followed by significant swelling, report them to your surgeon right away.

MOST COMMON RISKS & COMPLICATIONS OF COSMETIC PROCEDURES

General Risks

- Hematoma
- Seroma
- Skin sloughing (skin loss)
- Nerve damage (temporary injury to a nerve)
- Infection
- Bleeding
- Delayed healing

- Poor scarring or keloids (raised or hypertrophic scars)
- Prolonged numbness
- Reaction to anesthesia or medications (allergic reaction, nausea, vomiting)

Serious Complications

- Pulmonary embolus (a blood clot)
- Fat embolus
- Permanent nerve damage
- Malignant hyperthermia
- Arrhythmia
- Sepsis
- Death

How much does it cost?
Make sure that you are aware of all costs so there are no surprises.

ITEMIZED COSTS
Consultation fee
Surgical fee
Deposit
Anesthesia fee
Hospital or operating room charges
Photography
Medications
Laboratory fees
Implants
Surgical garments
Supplies and dressings
Nursing care

COSMETIC SURGERY FEES*

PROCEDURE	SURGICAL FEE RANGE
Rhinoplasty	$6,000 to $8,000
Abdominoplasty	$6,000 to $12,000
Bodylift	$10,000 to $14,000
Chin Implant	$2,500 to $4,000
Facelift	$5,000 to $15,000
Eyelidplasty or Browlift	$4,000 to $6,000
Breast Augmentation	$5,000 to $8,000
Breastlift or Reduction	$5,000 to $10,000
Armlift (Brachioplasty)	$4,000 to $8,000
Lipoplasty	$3,000 per area
Facelift, Eyelidplasty, Browlift	$15,000 to $25,000

* THESE FEES DO NOT INCLUDE ANESTHESIA, OPERATING ROOM, OR HOSPITAL FEES. AN ITEMIZED STATEMENT SHOULD BE PREPARED FOR YOU. COMBINING OPERATIONS IN ONE STAGE MAY REDUCE THE CHARGE PER PROCEDURE.

GETTING READY FOR SURGERY

What to Have on Hand

Ice

Food and beverages, especially water

A good friend

A babysitter

A dog walker

Take-out menus

Tylenol®

Arnica Montana for bruising

All prescription medications (pain medication, antibiotics) should be filled before the procedure

Essential medicine cabinet items including: extra bandages, antibacterial creams, topical medications, support garments, tissues, a thermometer

Any electronic items you cannot be without: phone, TV, laptop, portable music player, with extra chargers and batteries

CONTINUED

Extra blankets and warm covers
A heating pad
Three to four pillows propped (for facial procedures)
A stool softener (such as Colace® or Senokot®) taken the day before surgery can help with constipation.
Antibacterial soap; shower with antibacterial soap the morning of surgery
Loose, comfortable, breathable clothing is the best way to dress before and after surgery. For facial, breast or stomach procedures, wear loose button down or zippered shirts or robes (nothing that has to be pulled over your head)
Keep everything you need close at hand or in a bedside table

What to Avoid Before and After Surgery

Cigarettes If you are a smoker, stop for four to six weeks before surgery, or cut down on your smoking as much as possible. Many doctors will not perform surgery on a smoker, as tobacco can severely impact your healing and recovery.

Vitamins and Supplements Many vitamins can cause potential problems with your recovery. The safest approach is no vitamins for two weeks prior to your procedure.

Aspirin Avoid aspirin products such as Advil®, Motrin®, and Excedrin® as they may increase bruising. If you need to take a mild pain medication, take Tylenol®-based products only.

Nail polish Don't wear nail polish on the day of surgery. Doctors need to see your nail beds as part of their monitoring.

Valuables Leave all jewelry at home. It's one less thing to worry about.

Contact Lenses Don't wear contact lenses on the day of surgery. Bring your glasses if you need them.

Food No food or drink for at least eight hours before any procedure that requires anesthesia.

MEDICATIONS TO BE DISCONTINUED PRIOR TO SURGERY

THIS IS ONLY A PARTIAL LIST. CONSULT WITH YOUR DOCTOR BEFORE DISCONTINUING ANY MEDICATION.

ASPIRIN

Bufferin	Fiornal
Easprin	Darvon
Ecotrin	Lortab
Exedrin	Norgesic
Ascriptin	Aspergum
Alka Seltzer	

ANTI-INFLAMMATORIES

Advil	Anacin
Aleve	Empirin
Anaprox	Bufferin
Cataflam	Bayer
Clinoril	Entab-650
Dolobid	Indomethacin
Feldene	Indocin
Ibuprofen	Midol
Lodine	Nalfon
Ponstel	Relafen

ANTI-PYRETICS

Aleve	Trilisate
Feverall	

ARTHRITIS MEDICATIONS

Aleve	Dolobid
Anaprox	Ecotrin
Ansaid	Motrin
Cataflam	Indocin
Clinoril	Orudis
Daypro Solganal	Telectin
Voltaren	Mono-gesic

CONTINUED

Myochrysine	Ridaura
Sal-flex	Feldene
Lodine	Naprosyn
Oruvail	Toradol
Imitrex	Midrin
Blocadren	Migrilam
Ergomar	Wigraine
Ergostat	Fiorinal
Cafergot	Darvon
PLATELET INHIBITORS	
Aspirin	Halfprin
Baby Aspirin	Persantine
Bufferin	Ticlid
Ecotrin	
TOPICAL PREPARATIONS	
Absorbent Rub	Metholatum
Absorbine	Infrarub
Act-on-Rub	Solitice
Ben Gay	Oil-O-Sol
Doan's Rub	Panagesic
Exocaine Plus	Stimurub
Icy Hot	Surin
HEET	Yager's Lin.
Neurabain	Zemo Liquid
Sloan's	
COLD MEDICATIONS	
Alka-Seltzer	Quiet World Analgesic
Dristan	Sine-off
Vanquish	St. Joseph's for Children
Pepto-Bismol	

OTHER PRODUCTS CONTAINING ASPIRIN

ACA Caps	Empragen
APAC Acetonyl	Equagesic
Aidant	Excedrin
Alka Seltezer	Fiorinal
Allygesic	Fizrin
Apamead	Formasal
APC	Fizrin
Aphodyne	Formasal 4 way Cold Tabs
Aphophen	Gelsodyne
Arthra-Zene	Grillodyne
ASA	Hasamal CT
Asalco	Henasphen
Ascaphen	Histadyl
As-ca-phen	Hypan
ACD Acetabar	I-Pac
Acetasem	Kryl
Aprine	Liquiprin
Aluprin	Lumasprin
Amosodyne	Marnal
Amytal	Measurin
Anacin	Medadent
Amytal	Medaprin
Anexsia	Midol, Midol 200
Anadynos	Multihist
Ascodeen	Nembudeine
Ascriptin	Nembu-Gesic
Aspadine	Nipirin
Aspergum	Norgesic
Aspac	Novahistine
Aspencaf	Novrad

CONTINUED

Aspyte	Opacedrin
Aspirbar	Opasal
Aspir-C	Paadon
Aspireze	Pabirin
Aspirin (USP)	PAC
Aluminum	Palgesic
Children's Aspirin	PC-65
Aspircal	Pedidyne
Aspir-phen	Pentagesic
Axotal	Pentagill
Babylove	Percobarb
Bayer, Bayer Timed-Release	Percodan
Brogesic	Persistin
Bufabar	Phac Tab
Buff-A	Phenaphen
Buffacetin	Phencaset
Buff-a-comp	Phenergan
Buffadyne	Phenodyne
Bufferin	Pheno-Formasal
Buffinol	Phensal
Calurin	Pirseal
Cama Inlay	Palygesic
Capron	Ponodyne
Causalin	Predisal
Cephalgesic	Prolaire-B
Cheracol	Pyrasal
Cirin	Pyrhist Cold
Clistanal	Pyrroxate
Codasa	Phinex
Codempiral	Robaxisal
Codesal	Ryd
Coldate	Sal-Aceto

Colrex	Sal-Fayne
Congesprin	Emprazil
Cope	Salibar Jr
Coralson	Salipral
Modified Cordex	Sarogesic
Coricidin	Sedalgesic
Co-ryd	Semaldyne
Counter pain	Sigmagen
Covangesic	Sine-Off
Darvon, Darvon with ASA, Darvon Compound	Spirin Buffered
Davo-Tran	Stanback
Dasikon	Ster-Darvon
Dasin Caps	St. Joseph
Decagesic	Supac
Delenar	Super-Anahist
Derfort	Synalgos
Derfule	Synirin
Dolcin	Tetrex-APC
Dolene	Thephorin-AC
Dolor	Toloxidyne
Doloral	Trancogesic
Dorodal	Trancoprin
Drinacet	Triaminicin
Dristan	Trigesic
Drocogesic	Triocin
Duopac	Vanquish
Duradyne	Zactirim
Duragesic	Zorpin
Ecotrin	Feldene
Empiral	Indocin
Empirin	

Vitamins and Supplements

The following is only a partial list of oral supplements that should also be discontinued two weeks before and after surgery, as they may have the potential to interact with analgesics and anesthesia and can enhance the risk of bleeding:

- Vitamin E
- Echinacea
- Ginseng
- Garlic
- Gingko Biloba
- Bilberry
- Dong Kwai
- Feverfew
- St Johns Wort
- Ephedra
- Mah Huang
- Turmeric
- Meadowsweet
- Willow

CHECKLIST

- ☐ One word: CREDENTIALS.
- ☐ Get the facts from friends, patients, doctors.
- ☐ Do your homework on the Internet, and read some books about the procedure you are contemplating.
- ☐ Ask a million questions—and listen to the answers.
- ☐ Prepare yourself for surgery mentally, emotionally, and practically.

You should make sure that you have a personal rapport with your surgeon. Check your level of comfort with the doctor's staff , and see that you feel good about the level of communication you establish with them as well.

CHAPTER 2

The Quest for Cleavage

A Lustier Bustline

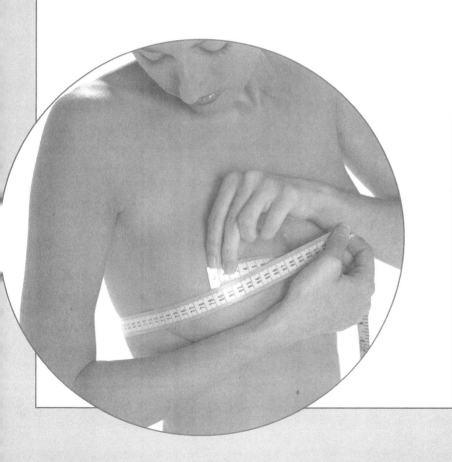

Every magazine on the newsstand confirms that beautiful, full breasts are the ticket to sex appeal. With models and actresses' cleavage getting higher and necklines getting lower, it is no surprise that breast augmentation is the third most popular procedure in the US. More and more younger women (between the ages of 18 and 24) are seeking cleavage. Breast implants are FDA-approved for women ages 18 and older, which means that almost any woman at any age can have cover girl cleavage.

Most Common Myths About Breast Augmentation

- **All breast implants can be felt to the touch.** In fact, most implants cannot be felt!

- **All breast implants harden over time.** Definitely, not true! Only about 15 percent of women develop hardening of scar tissue, called capsular contracture.

- **Silicone implants can cause cancer.** The highly-regarded Institute of Medicine dispelled possible links between illness and silicone implants! In 2006 the FDA repealed a 14-year ban.

BREAST AUGMENTATION

What's Hot
- Natural looking results
- Quick recovery
- Minimal or no visible scar
- Sub-pectoral placement
- Short surgery—less than one hour
- Minimal pain post-operatively

What's Not
- Fake-looking, surgically enhanced results
- Large, visible incisions
- Breasts that feel hard to the touch
- Above the muscle placement
- Long surgical times
- Anatomical implants

Benefits of Breast Augmentation
- A new and increased satisfaction with your breast size, shape and firmness
- A higher self-esteem
- Larger breasts which make your body look more proportional
- A reshaping of breasts that have lost their shape due to breast feeding, childbirth or age
- A balance in the appearance of breasts that once differed in size and shape

Breast augmentation is my favorite procedure. Women with breast augmentation are generally the happiest and are more excited about their results than those who undergo any other cosmetic surgical procedure.

In one study conducted by the Institute of Medicine, an impressive 95 percent of women said they would definitely choose to have the surgery again. This is certainly consistent with the feedback I hear from my patients on a daily basis.

The procedure has changed over the years because there are many newer types and shapes of implants available. The newest implants contain a cohesive silicone gel which does not leak. I believe breast augmentation is one of the most advanced and easiest procedures to perform and is therefore the safest for my patients. It can look natural, and provide beautiful results with minimal or no visible scarring. Breast augmentation is second in popularity only to liposuction, according to the American Society for Aesthetic Plastic Surgery.

I see more young girls now than ever before who are still growing into their bodies, but can't wait to have breasts like the hottest star on this week's edition of *US Weekly*. I have spoken to teens who came to see me with their parents because they are getting a new set of breasts as a high-school or college graduation present. The FDA approves saline breast implants for women ages 18 and over, but there are many reasons not to have breast augmentation at that age. To begin with, breasts start to develop during puberty in response to a flood of estrogen from the ovaries. The amount of fatty tissue that accumulates during puberty varies widely depending primarily on the response of each woman's body to estrogen. Sometimes the breasts respond very little and the amount of fatty tissue remains small; other times the breasts are overly sensitive to the hormone and an excessive accumulation of fat forms. The degree to which breast tissue reacts to hormones is an inherited trait.

During puberty, it is hard to predict exactly how your breasts will grow. Rapid growth may be followed by a period when you do not see much of a change. Sometimes one breast grows faster than the other, which would make any young woman feel incredibly self-conscious. For most women, breasts are not identical, but they do eventually become similar in size. In rare cases, only one breast develops fully. It makes sense to wait until your breasts are fully developed before considering breast augmentation. You need to be physically and emotionally ready for this kind of surgery, so if you are not sure, give your body a year or so to finish developing naturally. You can always make the choice to come in for surgery later.

GREENBERG'S LIST
Top Questions for Your Breast Augmentation Consultation

How long have you been doing breast augmentation surgery? At least three years is preferable.

How many breast augmentations do you perform each week? At least three is preferable.

What is the rate of reoperations needed? Your breast implants do not come with a lifetime guarantee and will need to be changed approximately every 15 years, but some patients can get a lifetime out of their implants.

What type of reoperation is the most common? Standard breast implant replacement is most common, usually for leakage from the valve.

Which incision method do you use? I prefer to place breast implants through a one and a half inch incision just under each of the woman's breasts. This makes for a very well-hidden scar.

Where do you place breast implants? In most cases, I prefer to place the implants sub-pectoral (under the chest muscle), rather than sub-glandular (under the gland). With saline-filled implants, the layer of muscle adds additional protection and helps to prevent the appearance of rippling or being able to feel the edge of the implant.

What types of implants do you prefer and why? I prefer a round, smooth implant because it offers the most natural look.

How do I know what my optimal breast size is? We will discuss your preferences and take into account your height, weight, and frame, as well as your lifestyle and level of physical activity, when determining your ideal breast size. Photographs often help to give a better idea of the result you are looking for. We also have implants in our office for patients to touch and try on by placing them inside your bra to get an idea of how a particular size will look and feel.

How long is the procedure? Should be at least about 35 to 40 minutes (but no more than one and a half hours for a routine breast augmentation.

What is the recovery like? Most patients experience some moderate discomfort for the first 48 to 72 hours. As the swelling resolves, the breasts will get soft and start to feel normal again.

How many operations on my implanted breasts can I expect over my lifetime? Expect a few, depending on your age when you first have the implants. Be wary of a surgeon who tells you this will be your only one.

How will my ability to breast feed be affected? In most cases, breast implants will not interfere with your ability to breast feed.

How can I expect my implanted breasts to look after pregnancy or breast feeding? Your breast skin will be stretched after pregnancies and breast feeding, but this should not affect the implant.

What are my options if I'm dissatisfied with the cosmetic outcome of my implanted breasts? You can have your implants removed, exchanged, or your breasts lifted, depending on your personal preferences.

Do you have before/after photographs? We have photographs to show you when you come in for your consultation.

SALINE VERSUS SILICONE FILLED IMPLANTS

The FDA now allows the use of both saline and silicone-filled breast implants manufactured by Mentor Corporation and Allergan Corporation. Silicone is approved for breast reconstruction but is limited for

cosmetic augmentation in women 22 and older. To date, all other
manufacturers' saline-filled breast implants are still being investigated.
Saline implants have a silicone rubber shell with sterile saline (salt
water) that is inflated to your desired size. Most implants have a valve
that is sealable by the surgeon. There are two types of saline-filled
implants. The most common type is a fixed volume implant, which
is filled with the entire volume of saline at the time of implantation.
Another type is an adjustable volume implant, which is filled in the
operating room, yet has the potential for further post-operative adjustment. The implants are filled with saline through a tube during surgery.
Since they are deflated when they are inserted, the surgeon is actually
placing a very small object inside you, which is one of the reasons the
incision can be tiny.

The Advantages

Saline implants have some advantages over silicone implants. Silicone
implant ruptures are harder to detect. When saline implants rupture,
they deflate and the results are seen almost immediately. When silicone
implants rupture, the breast often looks and feels the same because the
silicone gel may leak into surrounding areas
of the breast without a visible difference.
Replacing a ruptureds silicone gel implant
is more difficult than repairing a saline
implant. Silicone implants also have a higher
rate of capsular contracture (hardening of
scar tissue around the implant) and a higher
deflation rate. In addition, if a saline implant
rupture (which happens in less than four
percent of patients) it is completely safe.
Your body naturally absorbs the salt water.

Silicone implants have a silicone rubber shell that is filled with a fixed amount
of silicone gel. In the early 1990s it was reported that silicone breast
implants were responsible for Connective Tissue Diseases in some

What is capsular contracture?

Scar tissue forms around all implanted
materials as a natural part of healing.
Scar tissue around a breast implant is
not troublesome unless it tightens. An
abnormally tight scar is known as a
capsular contracture. This occurs in less
than 15 percent of cases, but this rate is
variable among patients from different
surgeons.

women. After a comprehensive evaluation, the Institute of Medicine concluded there was "no definitive evidence linking silicone breast implants to cancer, neurological diseases, neurological problems or other systemic diseases." Various silicones are used in lubricants and oils, as well as in silicone rubber. Silicone can be found in many common household items, such as polishes, suntan and hand lotion, antiperspirants, soaps, processed foods, waterproof coatings, and chewing gum. The FDA has approved many medical devices made of silicone, including replacement heart valves.

Dr. Greenberg's Most Requested Best Breasts

- Jessica Simpson
- Salma Hayek
- Giselle Bundchen
- Halle Berry

Some surgeons feel that silicone implants have a more natural look and feel than saline implants because silicone gel has a texture that is similar to breast tissue.

For more information about the safety aspects of breast augmentation, visit www.breastimplantsafety.org

SIZE, SHAPE AND TEXTURE OF BREAST IMPLANTS

Implants are available in three different shapes: round, breast shaped, and teardrop shaped. My preference is almost always round implants. The other shapes (known as anatomical implants) have many disadvantages when compared to the round implant. In my experience, the round implants look more natural than the anatomical implants. The anatomical implant can also shift or turn, which makes the breast look abnormal. Also available are smooth and textured implants. The textured implants tend to ripple more than the smooth, and in most cases, the textured implants offer no advantages.

High profile implants can be used for narrowly-framed women; mid-profile implants are the most commonly used because they provide for projection while sitting nicely in narrow breasts.

Just remember, it's important not to go too small! A common mistake women make is insisting upon an implant that is too small to provide optimal results. But the natural look is the way to go! Your surgeon should match breast implants to your own body type. Personalizing your breast implants is key!

Many women have no idea where to begin when choosing a new breast size. I will recommend the best size for you based upon your height, weight and frame. You can feel comfortable and confident listening to my advice as I have a lot of experience selecting the best implants for each individual patient. I will also evaluate your breast tissue to determine whether you have a sufficient amount to cover the breast implant. You may be surprised at what you can carry, and once you are comfortable with your new breasts, you may wish you had chosen the largest possible size appropriate to your physique. If you want a breast implant size that is too large for your tissue, I may warn you that breast implant edges may be visible after your surgery. Gravity also takes a toll on excessively large breast implants, resulting in premature drooping or sagging.

Your implant size is determined by the amount of saline inflating the implant. For instance, a 225 cubic centimeter (cc) implant means you are anticipating putting 225 ccs of saline into the implant. In some cases, I will overfill the implant by about 50 ccs; therefore a 225 cc implant may be inflated to about 275ccs. This is a relatively small implant, translating to approximately a small size-B. The most commonly used implant is a 350cc (or full C cup) implant. The final size of your augmented breasts is a combination of what you start with (your

Translating CC's to Cup Size

A cubic centimeter is a metric measurement of volume/capacity. According to a study conducted by the American Society of Plastic Surgeons, an average of 189cc of saline was needed to increase by one bra cup size. Increasing an A cup to a C cup required a total of 391cc, or 196cc per cup. Moving from a B cup to a D cup required a total of 448cc, or 224cc per cup. Every woman's body and breast size and shape is different, so these figures should only be used as a guide.

natural breast) plus the implant size. We can try to even out any asymmetries by using different amounts of saline or a different size implant.

Cup size can vary significantly among bra styles and manufacturers. We have implants in the office so that patients can try on different sizes by stuffing them inside their bra. Or you can try using plastic bags filled with oatmeal or rice to see how different sizes look in various types of clothing.

ABOVE OR BELOW THE CHEST MUSCLE—WHERE SHOULD YOUR IMPLANTS BE PLACED?

The breast consists of three parts: the inner cushion of milk-secreting glands embedded in fatty tissue, an outer envelope of skin, and the nipple/areola. The breasts rest atop the pectoral muscle that crosses the chest. Implants can be placed either underneath the chest muscle or on top of the chest muscle behind the soft fatty tissue.

In my opinion implants should be placed underneath the chest muscle for a number of reasons. First, this positioning enhances the ability to examine breasts for cancer using mammography. Second, it is the most natural and most attractive looking option. The implants are usually undetectable and they cannot be felt to the touch. Third, this method may reduce the occurrence of capsular contracture.

When implants are placed above the chest muscle, they sometimes appear "fake-looking." They also tend to "droop" more over time when placed above the muscle. The long-term explantation (removal) rate is much lower when the implant is placed under the muscle.

I almost always choose the short infra-mammary (under the breast) incision. This approach has several advantages. First, the incision is smaller than an inch, and is placed right underneath the crease of the breast. The scar heals exceptionally well and since it is hidden, it is virtually undetectable in the majority of patients. In addition, there is little chance of losing sensation in your nipples. I believe patients have the best long-term results and lowest overall complication rates using the crease incision.

Some surgeons elect to use the periareolar (around the nipple)

How do we insert breast implants?

- Through the armpit (transaxillary)
- Around the nipple (periareolar)
- Under the breast (inframammary)

incision. In this approach, an incision is placed around the bottom half of the areola and is usually very well concealed. The disadvantage of this approach is a higher risk of not being able to breast feed and/or losing nipple sensation. In addition, because the nipple is the focal point of your breast, any imperfection will be obvious. I almost never use the armpit incision because it is a more extensive procedure, requiring a longer recovery, and can leave a noticeable scar under your arm when you wear tank tops, bathing suits, or any strapless apparel.

Conquering the Consultation

When you are looking for a cosmetic breast surgeon, apply the same tips from Chapter One on how to find a plastic surgeon. Once you have chosen one or two doctors to visit, be sure you go to the consultation prepared, perhaps with your spouse or with another loved one who can provide an extra set of eyes and ears.

Your Surgery and Recovery

In most cases, I may suggest a mammogram before your procedure, and will also take pre-operative photographs. Often, the photographs are used in the operating room as another reference point. I sit my patients up during the procedure to ensure the breasts are properly aligned, have equal fullness, and generally look fantastic. The routine breast augmentation usually takes about 35 minutes (and no more than 90 minutes) to complete. It is generally an outpatient procedure, meaning you may go home the same day. I advise my patients to bring a loose, baggy zipper sweatshirt or button down shirt to wear home from the procedure.

Your chest will be bandaged for approximately 24 hours. After one day, we will take off your bandages and put you into a support strap for about three to four weeks. The strap helps the breasts settle into position. If you like, you can also wear a lightly supportive sports bra under the strap. You can wash and dry the strap in the laundry and take it off when you shower. You may also have little paper tapes (steri-strips) that cover the stitches. Leave these paper tapes alone; they come off by themselves in about one to two weeks. The stitches will likely be absorbable (meaning they dissolve on their own). You can shower after 24 hours and get everything wet, including the paper tapes—just pat them dry after the shower.

You will feel some tenderness following the procedure. Take your pain medication and muscle relaxants (if prescribed). You can also take Tylenol® every four hours. Sleep on your back or in a reclining position for the first few days following the surgery. Most women can return to work in a couple of days. You can return to all normal activities as soon as you feel comfortable. But there can be no exercising, running, or heavy lifting for four weeks. Be patient, the wait will be worth it!

About one week after the procedure, we will teach you a massage technique for your (smooth) implants. You may be massaging about three times per day for about two to three minutes each. The idea is to move the implants around in the pocket. This helps to soften them and decrease capsule formation. Squeeze the implant from the bottom to displace the implant upward, then squeeze from the top to displace it downward. Do the same thing from side to side. This displaces the implant out of its normal position and up into the excess pocket space above and on the sides.

One week after the procedure, I suggest taking vitamin E (400 IU) for about two months to help speed up the healing. (Some physicians feel that vitamin E may decrease capsule formation.) Women with textured implants should avoid implant exercises. A presumed advantage of the rough texture is that it allows surrounding tissue to stick to the implant, so as to prevent displacement. Performing implant exercise might negate this benefit by freeing the implant from surrounding soft tissue.

Congratulations! After the first week following the procedure, the hard part is over. Now you wait for the implants to settle, which takes up to three months. Initially the implants are high and hard. When the implants soften, they settle or drop into place. If they were placed where they looked perfect on the day you left the operating room, in two months your breasts would be too low. The implants are deliberately placed slightly higher to allow for the settling to occur. Don't worry, they will settle and you will soon love the results.

Will I need future breast operations?

The answer is a big maybe. Breast augmentation is a permanent procedure. The implants won't be absorbed by your body and they should remain in place forever unless you choose to have them moved. But they do sometimes deflate or cause other problems that significantly alter their appearance and require another surgery. If you have no such problems, your results should be long lasting.

Sources for more information....

Food and Drug Administration 1-888-INFO-FDA www.fda.gov/cdrh/breastimplants

Institute of Medicine Findings www.nap.edu/catalog/9618.html

Mentor Corporation 1-800-MENTOR-8 www.mentorcorp.com
Mentor also offers A Woman's Voice, which gives you straightforward advice from a nurse practitioner.

Allergan Inamed www.breastimplantstoday.com

TO LIFT OR NOT TO LIFT

If you are happy with your breast size, but are unhappy with what gravity, childbirth, or age have done to the shape of your breasts, then a breastlift (mastopexy) without implants may be right for you. As the skin loses its elasticity, the breasts often lose their shape and firmness and begin to sag. A breastlift raises and reshapes sagging breasts and can also reduce the size of your areola. We can achieve a lifted and fuller look by removing stretched or excess skin which causes the breasts to droop. Keep in mind that a breastlift won't keep you firm forever—the effects of gravity, pregnancy, aging, and weight fluctuations will eventually take their toll again.

Many women also choose to have implants with their breastlift. Women who have implants along with their breastlift may find the results last longer. Most women find that they look and feel better after a breastlift, both with and without clothes. Clothing and bras fit better. Women begin to break out the tiny tops and low cut dresses they never imagined they could fill out again.

Benefits of Breastlift

- Lifts sagging or droopy breasts
- Restores the contour of the breast after pregnancy or nursing
- Lifts the breast after loss of breast volume or weight
- Corrects asymmetries in the breast

THE DROOP FACTOR
To determine whether you need a lift, stand in front of your mirror and look at your nipples.

NO DROOP If your nipples point straight ahead, then you have no droop and do not need a breastlift.

MILD DROOP If your nipples have dropped to a level below the center of your breast but above your crease, then you have a mild droop.

MODERATE DROOP If your nipples have dropped below the crease of your breast, you have a moderate droop.

ADVANCED DROOP If your nipples have dropped below the crease and point downward, you have an advanced droop.

Whether you are concerned about wearing a skimpy outfit or what you will look like naked, visible scars are a valid consideration for women who want a breastlift.

Unlike breast augmentation, it can be difficult to hide the incisions of a breastlift procedure. A good rule of thumb is the greater the droop, the more extensive the incisions. Often, for only a small lift, the incision is made just around the areola with no other visible scars. This is an option for women whose breasts are fairly small and whose sag is minimal. For a complete breastlift in the patient who has significant loss of volume and droopiness, an incision that resembles an "anchor" shape is generally made.

Donut Incision

If you have small breasts you may be a candidate for the donut incision, in which a circular incision is made around the areola, and a donut-shaped area of skin is removed.

Lollipop Incision

The vertical lollipop is used if you require a "moderate lift." I will make an incision around the areola and straight down to the breast crease but not in the crease itself. This incision also "outlines" the breast area from which the skin is to be removed and "defines" the new location for your nipple. After excess skin is removed, the nipple and areola are moved to their new, higher position and the incision is closed, giving your breast a new contour.

Anchor Incision

The most common, an anchor-shaped incision, follows the natural contour of the breast, outlines the area from which breast skin will be removed, and defines the new location for the nipple. When the excess skin is removed, the nipple and areola are moved to a higher position. The skin surrounding the areola is then brought down and together to reshape the breast. Stitches are usually located around the areola, in a vertical line extending downward from the nipple area, and along the lower crease of the breast.

How We Do It

A breastlift can take anywhere from one to two hours. After surgery, you'll wear an elastic bandage or a surgical bra over gauze dressings. Your breasts will be bruised, swollen, and uncomfortable for a day or two, but the pain shouldn't be severe. Any discomfort you do feel can be relieved with medication.

Within a few days, the bandages or surgical bra will be replaced by a soft support bra. You'll need to wear this bra over a layer of gauze around the clock for three to four weeks. The stitches are usually absorbable.

If your breast skin is very dry following surgery, you can apply a moisturizer several times a day. Be careful not to tug at your skin in the process, and keep the moisturizer away from the suture areas.

You can expect some loss of feeling in your nipples and breast skin, caused by the swelling after surgery. This numbness usually fades as the swelling subsides over the next six weeks or so. In some patients, however, it may last a year or more, and occasionally is permanent.

Healing is a gradual process. Although you may be up and about in a day or two, don't plan on returning to work for about two to three days, depending on how you feel. And avoid lifting anything over your head for three to four weeks. If you have any unusual symptoms, don't hesitate to call your surgeon.

We will give you detailed instructions for resuming your normal activities. You may be instructed to avoid sex for a week or more, and to avoid strenuous sports for about a month. After that, you can resume these activities slowly. If you become pregnant, the operation should not affect your ability to breast-feed, since your milk ducts and nipples will be left intact.

Potential Pitfalls

Although the results can be positively life-altering, no surgery is a pleasurable experience, so you'll need to prepare yourself for the healing process. We will make every effort to make your scars as inconspicuous as possible. It is important to remember that mastopexy scars are extensive and permanent. They often remain lumpy and red for months, and then gradually become less obvious, sometimes eventually fading to thin white lines. Scarring is unpredictable and involves many factors including your own genetics, and family and medical history. Fortunately, the scars can usually be placed so that you can even wear low cut tops.

While there are no special risks that affect future pregnancies, pregnancy is likely to stretch your breasts again and offset the results of your procedure. So, if you are planning to have more children, it may be best to postpone your breastlift.

CHECKLIST

- [ ] Learn what is fact and fiction in breast augmentation.
- [ ] Silicone and saline implants each have their own unique benefits and drawbacks.
- [ ] Chose your uniquely appropriate breast size carefully after discussion with your doctor.
- [ ] Come prepared to ask your surgeon a slew of questions in the consultation.
- [ ] Know what to expect in surgery and beyond.

STRAIGHT FROM THE HEART

Tina is 40 years old, a divorced mother of four, and a small business owner.
Age: 40
Height: 5'7"
Weight: 134
Bra-size before implants: Small B
Bra-size after implants: Full D

"I always had nice breasts. I always liked the way they looked—until I started having kids. Then, they looked terrible. I was embarrassed by my appearance. I wouldn't even get undressed in front of my husband. After my second child, I knew I wanted breast implants. But I

decided to wait until after I finished having children. My husband didn't approve. He was very jealous. After I got separated, I was feeling down about myself and I decided to do something good for me. I found my doctor through referrals from a few of my customers. I saw their results and they looked wonderful. I went on one consultation and immediately felt comfortable with Dr. Greenberg. He was known for breast augmentation, and he knew exactly what I wanted done, so I did not feel the need to see anyone else. My breast augmentation was a great self-esteem tool. My body feels more balanced. I think I look more attractive. I get a lot of attention. I dress sexier and I don't hide my breasts—I flaunt them! I like the way they look and the way they feel. I have no regrets whatsoever. I am not ashamed. I don't hide the fact that I had breast augmentation. I love it! I would do it again no matter how much it hurt.

"I am very happy with the results! I went from a small size B-cup to a full size D-cup. When you lay down, they stand up straight. They don't flop to the side. When you're making love, you feel better, sexier. I buy so much lingerie now. I was so nervous about looking big and unnatural and disproportionate that I chose a smaller size than my doctor recommended. Dr. Greenberg originally said I should go bigger because I'm tall and I could carry it. Sure enough, after about six months, I did not think my breasts were full enough and so I went for an implant exchange to a larger size.

"Plastic surgery is just part of why I look good. I also do my work. I eat right and exercise five days per week. The older you get, the harder it is to stay in shape. Almost all of my friends want to have some kind of plastic surgery. I think they like the idea that I have had procedures done; it makes it more acceptable for them to make their own improvements. My advice is to make sure you are doing it for yourself and no one else. Choose your doctor by referral, make sure you know at least one person who went to him, and ask to see results.

"When it came to telling my four children, I took my time because I have two daughters, aged 13 and 15. They are at an impressionable

age and they watch everything you do. I wanted to be sure that they understood this was such an important decision for me, and not one to be taken lightly."

Dr. Greenberg's After Care

Sleep on two or three pillows for the first week following your procedure.

Leave your dressings intact until your surgeon sees you the next day to remove them.

You will be able to shower the day after the dressings are removed.

You will be placed into a surgical band. Wear this band under your clothes continuously for three weeks.

After three weeks you can wear a sports bra for an additional two to three weeks.

Your sutures are dissolvable and do not have to be removed.

Take the prescribed antibiotic until the prescription is completed.

Take your prescribed pain medication as directed.

Take Flexoril (muscle relaxant) for the first 48 to 72 hours only.

Do not take any aspirin or ibuprofen containing products for two weeks after your surgery. ONLY TYLENOL®.

No smoking for at least two weeks after you surgery

Start massaging one week after your procedure following Dr. Greenberg's method.

Do not lift any heavy objects or work out for four weeks after your surgery.

You must have an escort home, and someone to stay with you the night of surgery.

When your recovery is complete please be sure to follow up yearly with your primary care physician or Ob-Gyn for a yearly breast exam and mammogram.

CHAPTER 3

Losing Inches
with Liposuction

Smoother Contours

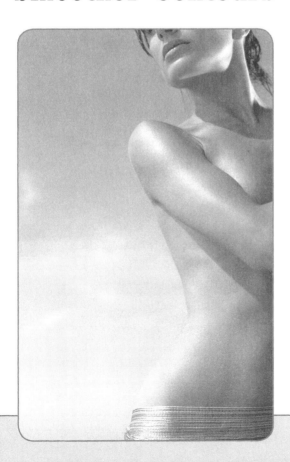

Almost all of us have a part of our body we would love to zap a bit of fat from. Even those of us who are close to our ideal weight often have problem areas that no amount of exercise and diet can eliminate. These fat deposits are often just handed down to us from our parents or grandparents. Women usually have the biggest complaints about their hips, thighs, and buttocks. Men find that fat collects around the stomach and love handles. Excess fatty deposits can also form around the chin, the arms, the back, and even the knees and ankles. Some things are beyond our control—such as the body we inherit and the effects of age. It's no surprise that liposuction is so popular; it allows you to take control of the uncontrollable, and it works!

What's Hot
- Quick recovery
- Little bruising and pain after surgery
- Top results, with fat and inches reduced dramatically
- Tiny, well-hidden incisions that leave virtually no visible scars

What's Not
- Using liposuction as a weight loss tool for obesity
- Removing more fat than is safe for the body and necessary for good results
- Expecting liposuction to get rid of cellulite. Liposuction removes fat cells, not cellulite. (VelaSmooth™ usually works for cellulite.)

BENEFITS OF LIPOSUCTION

1. Targets specific fatty deposits that are difficult to lose with diet and exercise
2. Permanently removes fat cells from your body
3. Helps provide a balanced, proportional look

Liposuction is the hottest cosmetic surgical procedure in the U.S. It can produce dramatic, life-changing results.

When we treat figure flaws such as pudgy hips and thighs with liposuction, we literally remove fat-storing cells. The more cells we remove, the less fat you will continue to develop in that area of your body.

GREENBERG'S LIST
Top Questions for Your Liposuction Consultation

How long have you been doing liposuction procedures? At least three years is preferable.

How many liposuction procedures do you perform each week? At least three is preferable.

What kind of results can I expect? Patient satisfaction with liposuction is extremely high, but we will talk about the specifics and address all of your concerns prior to surgery.

What techniques do you use and why? I use tumescent anesthesia. Some liposuction procedures are performed using ultrasonic energy or power assisted lipoplasty.

How long will the procedure take? It should be at least one hour for most liposuction procedures, slightly less for smaller areas, such as the chin, and can be up to three hours depending on the areas being treated.

Will I be bruised following the procedure and when will I see results? Most people do experience bruising and swelling following the procedure, which should begin to subside after about two weeks. You will begin to see results at about three weeks, which will continue to improve for at least six months following the procedure.

How much fat will you remove? The answer depends on your physique and desired outcome. In general, two to four liters of fat are removed during liposuction. More than five liters of fat and fluid is defined as a large volume liposuction requiring special safety precautions and an overnight hospital stay.

What is the average number of areas treated? Generally, anywhere from one to five areas is the norm—an area is defined as a particular section of the body such as hips, flanks, abdomen, inner and outer thighs, arms, etc.

How long does it take most of your patients to recover or return to work following liposuction? Most patients can go back to work over a long weekend from a small, limited liposuction. For larger volumes, up to five to seven days.

What is the likelihood of "touch up" or "refinement" procedures? It is not uncommon to have a small touch up after liposuction.

Liposuction was invented in 1978 in Paris by Yves-Gerard Illouz. Surgeons use a metal tube (cannula) about as wide as a pencil and a foot in length, and pass it through a small incision, usually in a natural crease of the skin. Because of the way the tool was developed, fat can be pulled through it without cutting into the other areas surrounding the fat cell. Fat cells are sucked out of the body, while the cannula rides over the arteries, nerves, and veins without damage. It is possible to remove a lot of fat with minimal blood loss and maintain a reasonably smooth contour. The tiny incisions made in liposuction virtually disappear, and once healed, most patients cannot even find where they were made!

The fat removed from the body is measured in liters (think of a liter-sized bottle of soda). In my opinion, five liters is the largest amount of fat that should be taken from the body during any one procedure in an outpatient surgery center. The average liposuction removes about two liters from the thigh and hip areas.

Liposuction definitely works. You will lose inches and fat. Most patients usually lose one or two pant sizes after liposuction of the thighs, hips, and buttocks. Just watch out for slick doctors who promise six-pack abs or the hips of a Victoria's Secret supermodel. Although "body sculpting" has become a popular catch phrase to describe liposuction, in essence, I believe the sculpting should only refer to the inch loss and fat loss. Liposuction isn't about chiseling or carving out new abs. If you're looking to shed those pesky pounds, liposuction isn't a miracle cure. While a maximum of about eight pounds (four liters) of fat can be removed, it is initially replaced with fluid from swelling, and most patients see very little immediate weight loss. Still, you will notice a dramatic change in your shape and the way your clothes fit.

The best candidate for liposuction is at a normal weight with localized problem areas of fat. The worst candidate is someone who is obese with poor skin tone. If you fall into this category, first try a safe, effective diet with the goal of losing as much weight as possible in a responsible way before having a liposuction procedure. If your skin is extremely lax, you may also benefit from skin removal, such as a tummy tuck or a thighlift.

Advances in liposuction, such as the tumescent and ultrasonic procedures, can give better results than were previously thought possible. I like to combine these procedures with traditional liposuction to remove the greatest amount of fat with the least amount of down time and post-operative recovery.

Am I a good candidate?

So you want to improve the contour of your body but you're still feeling pudgy even after years of diligent diet and exercise? If this sounds familiar, and you are at or close to your ideal body weight, liposuction may be for you. Liposuction can slim the hips and thighs, flatten the abdomen, and remove excess fat from the chin and upper arms. It can also help to create a shapelier contour of the inner knees, calves, and ankles. As long as you do not gain a lot of weight after surgery, the treated areas will maintain their contour!

Liposuction won't give you a flawless figure, so as with any cosmetic procedure, you need to keep your expectations realistic. There are certain areas of the body—such as the upper arms, abdomen, and inner thighs—which may develop loose or hanging skin following liposuction. The degree of skin retraction and tightness depends on age, the amount of fat to be removed, general skin tone, and degree of elasticity. If you are at high risk for loose skin, I may recommend a skin tightening procedure such as a thighlift, tummy tuck, or upper armlift. Sometimes noninvasive skin tightening procedures can be done such as Thermage® or ReFirme™. These use radiofrequency waves and can tighten skin in certain patients. Sometimes it is unclear whether you will develop loose skin after liposuction alone, but there is no need to panic: removal of excess or redundant skin can be performed at a later date.

What does liposuction do that a diet cannot?

When you diet, you shrink in weight and size, so specific areas of your body may look great. Liposuction reduces the overall number of fat cells in your body, which affects both the shape and contour. If you are only overweight in certain areas of your body, you would have to lose a larger amount of weight in order to shrink the size of your thighs. The weight will come off everywhere including the breasts and face, and not just where you need it most. From the face down to the ankles, most body parts can be suctioned for better contour and reduced volume. The most popular areas for women are the abdomen, inner thighs, outer thighs, hips, flanks, and knees. For those women with heavy breasts, liposuction can be used as an alternative to breast reduction.

While you may fantasize about draining every last drop of excess fat from your body, liposuction is not a miracle vacuum. As a rule, the liposuction of multiple areas should not exceed five liters of total fat removed in the outpatient setting and 10 liters in the inpatient setting. When large volume liposuction is performed, it is best to treat "aesthetic units" of the body to maximize the result. For instance, it is possible to combine liposuction of the back, love handle area, and abdomen during one session, and the hips, inner and outer thighs, and knees during another session.

How We Do It

The procedure is really simple. Tiny incisions of approximately less than one quarter inch long are made at the sites where fat is to be removed, and a wetting solution is infused to provide anesthesia, reduce bleeding, and improve fat extraction. This requires careful monitoring to avoid toxicity, and must be performed by those experienced with local anesthesia. We use various sizes and dimensions of cannulae—hollow, tubular instruments with holes at one end to trap the fat. The cannula is attached to suction tubing through which the excess fat is evacuated. I believe general anesthesia by an anesthesiologist is the safest way to perform liposuction. Local anesthesia alone for larger procedures can be dangerous.

These instruments come in various shapes, lengths, and sizes depending on the thickness and location of the fat. They have highly polished surfaces to slip through the fatty tissues with minimum friction or damage, and are frequently blunt-tipped to prevent cutting through the skin. Cannulae are inserted under the skin and are moved in a back and forth and criss-cross fashion within the fat, essentially pushing it aside while protecting the vessels and nerves. Fat is suctioned out through one or several holes at the tip, measured, and then the patient is checked for symmetry. The procedure is completed when a safe level of fat removal and the desired contour has been achieved. We closely monitor you to make sure that enough fluid hydration has been received. I use very small cannulae to mold and sculpt with greater accuracy and obtain overall better results.

Superwet Technique

The "wet" techniques and the superwet technique, referring to the amount of fluids injected, are variations of the tumescent technique. Tumescent anesthesia has had perhaps the most significant impact of all developments in liposuction. Warmed tumescent liquid—a diluted solution containing lidocaine, epinephrine and intravenous fluid—is injected into the area to be treated. As the liquid enters the fat, it becomes swollen, firm, and blanched. The expanded fat compartments allow the liposuction cannula to travel smoothly beneath the skin as the fat is removed. The saline softens the fat, the adrenaline decreases the blood loss and bruising, and the anesthesia provides relief from discomfort. Tumescent liposuction improves results and minimizes risks.

For small amounts of fat, the tumescent solution may be the only anesthetic given, or it can be supplemented with sedatives to put you in a sleepy state.

ADVANTAGES OF THE TUMESCENT TECHNIQUE
Quicker recovery: Within a short time after the procedure, patients can get up and walk out of the office, and they return to their regular routine within one week
Significantly less post-operative discomfort
Less bruising
Minimal scarring
Minimal trauma

Ultrasound Assisted Liposuction (UAL)

Ultrasonic sound waves, like shock waves, are transmitted into the fatty tissues from the tip of the cannula probe. The fat cells are melted or liquefied and then removed by low-pressure vacuum through a suction tube. Ultrasonic liposuction is often reserved for more difficult areas to contour where the deep fat is thicker, and thus harder to extract, i.e. back rolls, upper abdomen (as in male breast enlargement or gynecomastia), and flanks. It can be combined with traditional liposuction when both the deeper fat and more superficial fat are being removed. Some physicians use external ultrasound with liposuction in lower frequencies to soften fat deposits from the skin's surface. The literature shows limited effects of this treatment except on the tissues just below the skin surface. UAL can have a higher complication rate and I don't think that it is necessary in most patients.

Dr. Greenberg's Most Requested Lethal Legs

- Uma Thurman
- Gisele Bündchen
- Hilary Swank
- Cameron Diaz
- Naomi Campbell

Power Assisted Lipoplasty (PAL)

One of the latest advances in technology for liposuction is the addition of power. The cannulae used are motor-driven so they vibrate, which makes removing fat easier and faster for the surgeon. The primary advantage is that there is less physical exertion required to remove the fat with this method and therefore, sculpting of the fatty bulges is more controlled. In my opinion, it offers no significant benefit to you, the patient.

What to Expect Afterward

Depending upon the location and the amount of areas to be treated, the liposuction procedure usually takes between one and two hours. Liposuction can safely be performed with other cosmetic procedures, such as breast augmentation, eyelid surgery, or nose surgery. You can go home the same day of the procedure, and many patients can return to work after four days.

For large volume procedures over five liters, you may want to stay overnight in the hospital. You will probably experience some discomfort for about three days. Although you will feel fine, you will be bruised and swollen for about three weeks. Most patients say they feel like they worked out in the gym for a day or so after liposuction and don't have significant pain.

You have only one stitch in each incision. Some oozing for 12 to 24 hours is very normal. We use a large amount of fluid in the area in order to decrease the post-operative bruising and the discomfort. This fluid which mixes with a small amount of blood oozes out for the first day or so. The garment that you will be wearing is important to help decrease the bruising and swelling. Take the garment off to shower the next day. You can use any type of soap, and just pat the incisions dry after the shower. You do not need any further bandages, and you will not need to cover the incisions. Wash the garment and dry it while in the shower. It is fine to be without the garment for short periods of time, and it will not affect the result.

You will wear a support garment for about four weeks. During the first two weeks, you should wear the garment around the clock, only taking it off when you shower. If you only had your legs done, you can switch over to tight bicycle pants at about two weeks. For the last two weeks, I recommend you wear the garment for 12 out of 24 hours.

You will weigh more right after liposuction than before surgery, but there is no need to worry. Your face, feet, and hands may swell up from all the fluids given during the procedure, and the swelling is only temporary. Swelling travels down toward the feet with gravity, so it is not uncommon to be bruised and swollen in places where liposuction was not performed. There will also be numbness in some areas. Many people can return to work or limited activity within two days, and resume an exercise program to whatever degree they can tolerate in four weeks.

It takes a long while to see great results after liposuction. It is a slow process. Some areas you just can't get rid of because it is extra skin, muscle, or the fat and is not accessible to liposuction. You can see your new shape best after six weeks when most of the swelling has subsided. Residual swelling settles and skin tightens gradually over the next three to six months. You will begin to see your results once the bruising and swelling start to disappear. The results will continue to improve for several months. In most areas of the body, your skin will redrape itself against your new physique, leaving you with a beautiful, smooth contour.

A major benefit of liposuction surgery is that the scars are small and usually located in inconspicuous areas.

You will feel soreness and discomfort today, this is very normal. By tomorrow, a lot of your discomfort will be gone. Take the antibiotics that you were prescribed until they are finished. Continue to take iron and vitamin C for about a week. (It's probably a good idea to take a stool softener with it). You can resume any other vitamins in three or four days. Take your pain medications if you have a lot of pain. I find it better to take one pain pill with one Tylenol® unless you are having extreme discomfort, then take two pain pills. You can do whatever you feel comfortable doing. I want you up and around, and I want you to drink a lot of fluids for the first two or three days. It is very important to keep yourself very well hydrated, (water, juices, and sports drinks are best). No working out in the gym for four weeks.

The small slit-like openings for the liposuction cannulae can be placed in hidden areas like the upper skin fold of the navel, in the crease under the buttocks, and inside the knee, so they are well concealed. These scars generally heal well and usually do not pose a problem.

Potential Pitfalls

In rare situations, the tumescent technique can cause complications like pulmonary edema, which is a collection of fluid in the lungs that may occur if too much fluid is administered. Another potentially fatal complication can arise from lidocaine toxicity which can occur when a large amount of solution containing lidocaine is used. This is rare because I use low levels of lidocaine and general anesthesia. Anti-embolism boots are often used during surgery to prevent a blood clot from forming in the deep veins of the pelvis or legs. If a clot forms, the thigh or calf gets tender and the ankles swell. If this clot breaks free and travels to the lungs, there is a danger that it will impair breathing. A fat embolus can also occur where a bit of fat travels through the bloodstream and into the lungs, blocking breathing. A fluid collection called a seroma can develop especially after the ultrasound technique, and is more common in the abdomen and male chest area. In rare cases, I may need to drain the excess fluid in the office to relieve pressure. High volume liposuction procedures in which a large volume of fat is removed involve greater risks.

In some cases, a touch up may be done six months after the initial procedure to refine an area that has previously been treated. A small touch-up procedure to fix under treated areas is performed in about ten percent of patients six months later. The results of liposuction are permanent, as long as you keep your weight stable. If you gain weight after liposuction, you will tend to gain it back uniformly throughout the body since the normal number of fat cells are still there and will continue to expand. There are still fat cells in the areas that were suctioned. If you do gain fat in other areas of the body that were not your primary trouble spots, your body will usually be very responsive to diet and exercise. Because most of the fat cells are removed from the areas where we perform liposuction, it is rare for the fat to return to the areas that we liposucted.

Although liposuction is an effective method for removing fat deposits, it does not cure cellulite, tighten loose skin, or affect the fat that lies underneath the muscle layer. When the degree of skin elasticity is not easy to assess, a staged procedure may be effective. Liposuction can be used to contour the legs from the ankles, calves, and knees up to the inner and outer thighs, taking inches off the circumference of the leg. Calves and anterior thighs are tricky because they are often largely muscle, but suctioning even small amounts can make a big difference in the overall shape. Liposuction of the legs may take longer than other areas to fully settle down because swelling tends to travel downward and rest below the knee.

When it comes to liposuction, the tighter your skin, the better result you will have. If you have loose skin due to pregnancies, aging, or weight fluctuations, liposuction can potentially make the treated area look worse. Some areas of fat deposits are less forgiving than others, and more often lead to sagging skin: upper arms, inner thighs, abdomen, and the neck. The flanks and outer thighs are areas that respond very well after liposuction, and it is less common to develop loose skin in these areas. If your ultimate goal is to be taut, a tummy tuck, thighlift, or lower bodylift—which involves tightening underlying muscles and removing and redraping excess skin—are the only viable options. The trade-off is that the scars may be visible, and the recovery period is considerably longer than with liposuction alone.

NON-SURGICAL FAT REDUCTION

There is a new category of devices that is exploding onto the market that use ultrasound to treat localized fat deposits without making an incision. These devices (LipoSonix®, UltraShape™) may be best used for recontouring bulges rather than large volume fat removal. At the time of this printing, these devices have not yet received FDA clearance for marketing in the US. However, UltraShape™ is expected to be available in 2007.

LIPOTHERAPY

Another technique, the injection of phosphatidylcholine, a derivative of lecithin, is also being used to dissolve fat without the need for surgical intervention. This is done by injecting the area to reduce fat accumulations, and multiple treatments are needed. Injection lipolysis is exclusively concerned with achieving aesthetic improvements in body shape by dissolving small, defined zones of fat in problem areas. Claims as to the safety and efficacy of this product have so far not been substantiated by scientific clinical trials in the United States, but this method is widely used in Europe with some success.

Targeting Cellulite

Cellulite is caused by numerous factors including poor circulation and fibrosis of surrounding tissue. The main cause, however, is female hormones such as estrogen. Any combination of these leads to the rippled appearance and cold feel of the skin. Treatments vary according to the stage of cellulite being treated. There is no cure for cellulite, but effective treatments are now available.

Liposuction removes fat, but it does nothing for the rippled lines of dreaded cellulite. These dimpled fat deposits—usually around the hips, thighs, and buttocks areas—affect men and women. If you have cellulite before your liposuction procedure, you will have cellulite after the procedure.

What are the stages of cellulite?

Stage 1 Skin is cool to the touch, and presence of spider veins.

Stage 2 Dimpling of the skin present when pinched.

Stage 3 Cellulite is visible when standing but disappears when you lay down.

Stage 4 Cellulite is visible when standing and does not disappear when you lay down.

Endermologie®

I recommend Endermologie® (LPG) following liposuction for patients who are trying to complete their gorgeous new body by getting rid of cellulite. Endermologie® is a very effective cellulite reduction treatment that uses rollers and suction to improve your skin's tone and condition. Endermologie® feels like a deep massage. In addition to its cosmetic benefits, the therapeutic benefits include an improvement in your overall blood and lymph circulation. We recommend a minimum of six to ten Endermologie® sessions for best results. The weekly sessions generally last about 35 minutes.

VelaSmooth™ Radiofrequency Waves

VelaSmooth™ (Syneron) improves local circulation and will give your skin a smooth, contoured appearance. VelaSmooth™ treatments are unique because different maneuvers are used to reach different layers of tissue and fat. In combination with the maneuvers, suction and rollers gently lift the skin. All areas of the body can be easily treated. The VelaSmooth™ treatments are individualized to each patient, depending on the areas that need the most attention. VelaSmooth™ can also be combined with liposuction to help smooth out problem areas which will not respond to diet and exercise. We recommend 16 treatment sessions, which are 30 minutes each. When your treatments are finished, one session per month is recommended to maintain your results.

STRAIGHT FROM THE HEART

Donna is a single woman who works as an office manager. She had liposuction on her inner and outer thighs about six and a half months before this interview.

Age: 26
Height: 5'6"
Pants size before Liposuction: Size 10
Pants size after Liposuction: Size 6

"I never even thought about plastic surgery until I ran into a friend who had liposuction, and she looked great. When I first met her, she was wearing these black Guess jeans (I have the same pants), and I remember thinking, 'Wow, she is gorgeous, but her ass is huge!' When I saw her after the procedure, she looked so good that she inspired me to do something about my own body. Even so, it took me about two years after I saw her to get the courage to have liposuction myself.

"When I went in for my consultation, I made it clear to Dr. Greenberg what I wanted done. I think looking at before/after photos is a good idea, even if the practice definitely just picks their best patients for their books.

"After the procedure, I was really bruised and really swollen and I couldn't see the results right away. My mom didn't want to see my

legs, and she wouldn't even look at my bruises. In fact, she probably didn't look at my legs for about three months. Then, I showed her my results and she saw me in my clothes. I gave all my pants to her because they didn't fit me any more. When she saw my results, she couldn't believe it. Now she wants to have something done! My boyfriend, who supported by from the beginning, loves the results. He says, 'You honestly do look so much better.' My figure is so much more proportionate now. Doctor Greenberg took out two liters of fat (one from each leg), which is a lot of fat, like a two-liter bottle of soda.

"I had about five treatments of Endermologie® after the liposuction (doctor recommended). After lipo, you're very hard and numb. The Endermologie® brings your feeling back and loosens everything up, so you're not tight. It must improve your circulation. It feels really good. I would definitely tell everyone to get Endermologie® after liposuction. It minimizes cellulite and speeds up the heeling process.

"Dr. Greenberg did a great job. I'm much thinner now. My legs are totally even. I have absolutely no scars that anyone can see, which I think is great. I had liposuction on a Thursday night. I was up and around immediately, but by Sunday I was really feeling better. I went back to work on Monday. I would definitely do it again, no doubt about it! My friends see how happy I am with the results and they are following suit!"

CHECKLIST

☐ Liposuction is not a weight loss tool or a cure for cellulite.

☐ Liposuction can improve your body's contour and create a more proportional look.

☐ Swelling and scarring are to be expected and will subside over time.

☐ Liposuction will not confine you to bed rest—you will be up and back to yourself in a matter of days.

☐ View liposuction realistically. It is not a cure-all or a guarantee that fat will never return.

☐ Endermologie® and VelaSmooth™ can be used as a complementary procedure to noticeably smooth out cellulite after liposuction.

DR. GREENBERG'S AFTER CARE

You will be provided with medication for relief of pain.

You are allowed to drive 48 hours after surgery but should not drive if you have recently taken sedatives, narcotics, pain medications, or if you have significant pain.

Smoking and drinking alcohol are not recommended for two weeks after surgery.

Do not bathe or remove your support garment for the first 48 hours after surgery. You may shower 48 hours after the surgery.

Some bloody drainage may be seen. This is normal. Any bleeding or bruising that appears excessive should be brought to the attention of Dr. Greenberg immediately.

Wear your support garment continuously for the first two days after surgery. After this, you may remove the garment to shower.

You are encouraged to perform daily activities as tolerated 48 hours after surgery. You may start working out three to four weeks after the surgery.

Do not take ibuprofen or aspirin for two weeks following your procedure.

Take the prescribed antibiotic until the prescription is complete.

CHAPTER 4

The Allure of Flat Abs

Less Invasive Tummy Tucks

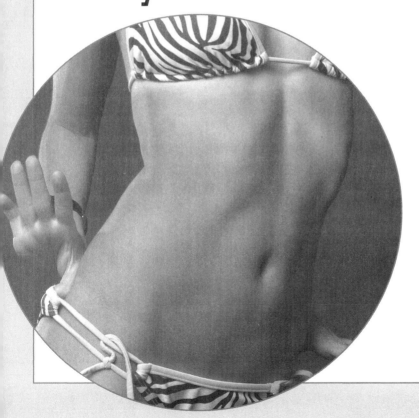

What's Hot
- Getting the stomach you've always dreamed of
- Reshaping your waist to improve contours
- Skin removal and tightening after multiple pregnancies

What's Not
- Going for a tummy tuck if you are not finished having children, unless you are not planning on having children anytime soon
- Thinking of tummy tuck surgery as a first resort rather than a last, after diet and exercise

M any women wonder whether they should have liposuction or abdominoplasty (a tummy tuck) to achieve their goal of a flat abdomen. Abdominoplasty, commonly known as a "tummy tuck," is a body contouring technique to remove excess skin and fat from the middle and lower abdomen and to tighten the muscles of the abdominal wall. The waistline also becomes better defined and a large, floppy navel, or one that has the appearance of a frown, can be converted into a small elliptical navel. Stretch marks and old scars that are located below the navel can be removed if they are part of the abdominal wall tissue that is discarded.

The best candidates for a tummy tuck are in relatively good shape, with loose abdominal skin. If there is a large fat accumulation on the abdominal wall, especially along the upper part, liposuction may be required at a second stage after an abdominoplasty removes loose skin and tightens muscles. Liposuction can also be performed as a primary procedure before abdominoplasty to debulk the fatty layer. Both a partial and complete abdominoplasty may be performed in conjunction with limited liposuction to remove fat deposits from the hips, waist, or thighs for a better contour. Extensive liposuction or multiple areas of treatment should be avoided at the time of tummy tuck as the surgical risks increase when these procedures are combined.

Women whose abdominal muscles and skin have been stretched

out from multiple pregnancies, as well as older women who have a loss of skin elasticity due to age or weight fluctuations, are excellent candidates for abdominoplasty. I often advise women who are planning future pregnancies to wait, as the vertical muscles in the abdomen that are tightened during surgery will tend to separate again during pregnancy.

Men are also candidates for abdominoplasty following massive weight loss or due to aging and lack of exercise. If your fat deposits and loose skin are all located below the navel, a less complex procedure called a mini-tummy tuck or partial abdominoplasty may be recommended.

GREENBERG'S LIST
Top Questions for Your Tummy Tuck

How long have you been doing abdominoplasty procedures? At least three years is preferable.

How many abdominoplasty procedures do you perform each week? At least two is preferable.

What kind of results can I expect? Patient satisfaction is extremely high, and in many cases, a flat abdomen is possible to achieve.

What techniques do you use and why? I perform liposuction, full abdominoplasty and mini abdominoplasty, depending on the amount of skin and fat present and the desired contouring.

How long will the procedure take? Depending on the extent of the procedure, two to four hours is typical.

Will I be bruised following the procedure and when will I see results? You will have moderate bruising for two to three weeks, and soreness that medication will help to alleviate. Swelling and discomfort is to be expected, and it may take three to six weeks to see your results.

How long does it take most of your patients to recover or return to work? Most people are able to return to work after 10 to 14 days.

What is the likelihood of "touch up" or "refinement" procedures? As a tummy tuck is an open procedure, touch ups are usually not necessary.

How We Do It

There are three basic approaches to contouring the abdomen, depending on your goals and the amount of skin, fat and muscle that needs to be addressed.

- Liposuction only
- Mini abdominoplasty
- Full abdominoplasty

Liposuction Only

For some patients, we can use liposuction alone to achieve a slimmer contour of the abdomen, flank and hip region. Liposuction can be performed alone or in combination with skin tightening procedures. Tummy tucks are often performed with liposuction of the hips and thighs and thighlifts are complemented by liposuction of the hips and abdomen.

Dr. Greenberg's Most Requested Awesome Abs:

- Jessica Alba
- Demi Moore
- Janet Jackson
- Christina Aguilera

Mini Abdominoplasty

The lowest part of the abdomen just below the belly button is subject to laxity. Here the rectus muscles only have an outer layer of fascia. Pregnancy and weight fluctuations stretch the abdominal wall and it doesn't always shrink back to its original state. This leads to permanent stretching. A mini-tummy tuck is designed for cases where the muscle wall laxity is restricted to this lower abdomen only. If there is less extra skin to be removed, I can sometimes use a smaller incision to redrape the remaining tissue of the abdominal wall. The smaller incision provides adequate access to repairs of the lower muscle wall. Excess fat can be removed with liposuction to enhance the contour.

Surgery can involve more extensive sculpture of the abdominal muscle wall. To get to the upper muscle wall from below, the belly button connection to the muscle wall needs to be elevated. I can place it in the same position or move it down as needed. When the bellybutton is lowered, upper abdominal skin can be tightened as well.

If you have a small degree of excess skin below the navel, a mini-tummy tuck may be all that is needed. In partial or modified tummy tuck, the incision is much shorter and the navel may not need to be moved. The skin is separated only between the incision line and the navel. This skin flap is stretched down, the excess is removed, and the flap is stitched back into place. Most post-pregnancy women have stretched out muscles and excess skin above the navel. With a limited abdominoplasty surgery, I can contour excess skin and fat below the belly button. This is a common site of loose extra tissue especially after pregnancy. The incision is usually smaller for the mini abdominoplasty. Abdominal muscles can be tightened through the incision. However, the mini tuck does not manage as much excess skin as does the standard abdominoplasty. The best candidates will have small amount of excess skin only below the navel and have otherwise firm abdominal muscles. This operation is best suited for cases that are not severe enough to need a full abdominoplasty, yet are too extensive for liposuction alone.

In some cases, limited incision mini abdominoplasties may leave excess skin on either end of the incision site which gives the appearance of what is referred to as "dog ears." It is not ideal for all women, but my patients usually want to try to avoid a longer scar and more extensive recovery whenever possible.

Full Abdominoplasty

For people who have more skin laxity or excess skin, a traditional tummy tuck is the best method to produce a flat abdominal contour. A tummy tuck is nearly always performed under general anesthesia. The most common technique involves an incision made across the lower abdomen, just above the pubic area, extending to the hip on each side. This incision can be angled higher or lower to make it easier to conceal, depending on whether low rise pants or high cut bikinis are more desirable. A second incision is usually made to free the navel from surrounding tissue. We then separate the skin from the abdominal wall all the way up to your ribs and lift a large skin flap to reveal the vertical muscles in your abdomen. These muscles are tightened by pulling them close together and stitching them into their new position. The skin flap is then stretched down and the extra skin and attached fat is removed. A new opening is made for your navel that has remained in the same position. The incisions are closed with dissolvable sutures, and surgical tape is placed over the incisions followed by a gauze dressing. It is not safe to aggressively liposuction the love handles (flanks) at the time of a tummy tuck. Sometimes we need to do future liposuction about three to four months after a tummy tuck. I often will use a "pain pump" which limits the amount of post-operative discomfort.

What Can I Expect After Surgery?

You will have soreness that can be controlled with medication. The morning after surgery, the dressing will be replaced with an abdominal supporter that you will be instructed to wear for several weeks. Drains are usually placed beneath the abdominal skin flap to collect small amounts of blood and serous fluid that may be secreted. The drains are easily removed in the office about five to seven days after the surgery.

While in bed the legs should be bent at the hips in order to reduce the strain on the abdominal area. You will be up and around the day of surgery, but it is important to avoid heavy lifting or exercise for three or four weeks. Most people are able to return to work after 10 to 14 days.

At first you may not be able to stand up straight without feeling a tugging sensation, but you should start walking as soon as possible as your body accommodates to your newly tightened abdomen (usually three to four days). Post-operative bruising is minimal, but swelling may take up to three months to a year to settle. You may also experience a loss sensation of the abdominal skin that may take several months to a year to return (sometimes the numbness is permanent). Surface stitches, if used, will be removed in five to seven days, and deeper sutures will dissolve on their own. (I use almost exclusively absorbable sutures.) Lighter bandages will be applied that will be replaced with an abdominal support garment that is worn for several weeks. Vigorous exercise should be avoided until you can do it comfortably, at about four to six weeks. It may take nine months to a year before the scars completely flatten, soften and lighten, but it may be sooner in fair skinned individuals (scarring is always variable and unpredictable in cosmetic surgery).

The recovery will be shorter with a mini-tuck procedure, and scar is about the same length as a C-section scar. Most patients are up and about in four to seven days.

Potential Pitfalls

Abdominoplasty surgery usually requires general anesthesia. In most cases, we can perform a tummy tuck on an outpatient basis. Since this procedure addresses skin, fat and musculature, it is more extensive than liposuction.

Possible complications include infection, bleeding, poor scarring, skin loss, asymmetries, the need for a revision, and others. This surgery does produce a permanent scar, which can extend from hip to hip in a full tummy tuck. In some cases, the scar may be thick, raised and irregular. Occasionally, a projection of bulging tissue on the ends of the scar called a "dog ear" can result which can be easily revised at a later date if necessary. Infections are rare, but when they occur, they can be treated with drainage and antibiotics. The risk of blood clots can be minimized by moving around as soon as possible after surgery. Poor healing, which results in conspicuous scars, may necessitate a second operation. Smokers have an increased risk of tissue loss and delayed healing. Nerves to the lower parts of the abdominal wall are divided when redraping the skin. There are often areas of the abdominal skin that will be numb after surgery. Although there is some risk for permanent numbness, this is quite rare.

STRAIGHT FROM THE HEART

Stephanie is a mother of two, and a former fitness instructor.
Age: 32
Height: 5'5"
Size before tummy tuck: 6
Size after tummy tuck: 4

"I used to be an aerobics instructor, so I always took great care of my body and was in super shape all my life. Then, I had kids and I started to notice that my tummy would not tighten back up, no matter how many crunches I did. I tried a few diets, drank a ton of water, and worked out with a trainer. But I did not see the results. I was frustrated. I just was not used to having so little control over how I looked!

"A girlfriend of mine who had just had a baby was really excited about her tummy tuck after having a baby. She was a thin, attractive woman, but she was very self-conscious about the loose skin on her lower abdomen. She was done having kids, so she was comfortable going in for surgery.

"I decided to take matters into my own hands, so I went in for a series of consultations and really loved Dr. Greenberg. He was confident but very sensitive to my insecurities and concerns. I scheduled my surgery while my kids were away at summer camp because I wanted to give myself time to heal, and I did not want them to see me afterward, in case I was in a lot of pain.

"I was able to get back to my normal daily activities within the first few days after surgery. I was sore, swollen and bruised, but I could still walk around and get things done. I was more excited to see the final result. Once the swelling went down, and the scars began to fade, I was so happy that I forgot all about the discomfort. I definitely recommend a tummy tuck to any woman who wants to get her pre-baby body back. My husband is happy because I am more confident about my looks, and I feel so much more attractive. There

is no reason to feel like you cannot take control of your body, look as great as you did ten years ago, and still be a mother!"

CHECKLIST

☐ Abdominoplasty is great for tightening and smoothing out skin after pregnancy or major weight loss

☐ Liposuction can be used alone or with abdominoplasty recontour the waist, hips and thighs

DR. GREENBERG'S AFTER CARE

Sleep with head elevated, and knees bent at all times for one week.

Walk bent over to avoid putting stress on your abdominal sutures.

Leave the dressing intact. Your doctor will see you on post-operative day number one and change dressings.

You will be able to shower 48 hours after surgery, with your drains in place. Remove all dressings and binder and shower, your drains can get wet.

Empty drains every 12 hours. Record the amount of drainage from each drain every 12 hours. If the drainage becomes excessive or drastically increases, call the office. Drains will be removed in approximately five to seven days, when drains are at minimum. Both drains will not be removed on the same day.

Most of your sutures will dissolve on their own.

Take the prescribed antibiotic until the prescription is completed. You must remain on antibiotics until all drains are removed.

Take your prescribed pain medication as directed.

Do not take any aspirin or any ibuprofen for three weeks after your surgery.

Take either stool softeners, prune juice or milk of magnesia. Start one day after surgery. If severe constipation occurs take milk of magnesia twice a day along with the stool softener.

Wear your binder for four weeks after surgery. You can use a panty girdle after one week.

Do a lot of deep breathing to expand your lungs. Do not become sedentary, ambulate as tolerated.

CONTINUED

No smoking for at least four weeks after your surgery.

Start with liquids and light food and advance your diet as tolerates.

Do not lift any heavy objects for the first 14 days after your surgery.

No heavy physical activity for four to six weeks.

Call the office if severe abdominal pain, fevers, redness of incisions, excessive drainage, or any other concerns.

CHAPTER 5

Bringing Up the Rear

Trends in Bodylifting

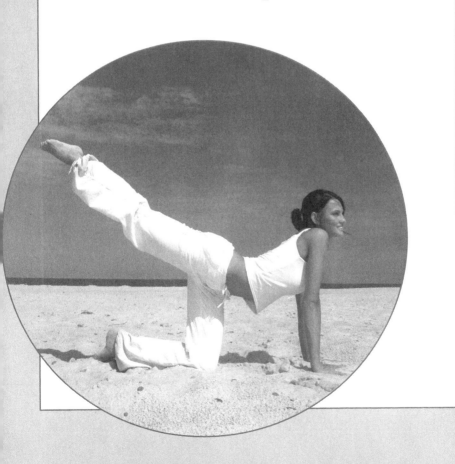

What's Hot
* Massive weight loss from disciplined diet and exercise
* Rediscovering the shape you had years ago—and flaunting it
* Staging several body contouring procedures to create a more symmetrical result

What's Not
* An unhealthy weight that can contribute to serious medical conditions and quality of life
* Loose, hanging skin that won't go away
* Ignoring post-surgery guidelines—they are there for your benefit!

K udos to anyone who has lost a large amount of weight (say more than 75 pounds)! You have accomplished a difficult goal. Now your years of struggling and failed diets are behind you. Perhaps you did it through weight loss surgery. Or, perhaps it was the more traditional way, through diet and exercise. However you did it, you deserve a new body as a reward for all your hard work.

GREENBERG'S LIST
Top Questions for Your Bodylift

How long have you been doing bodylift procedures? At least three years is preferable, but this procedure has become much more popular in the last few years.

How many bodylift procedures do you perform each week? At least one to two is preferable.

What kind of results can I expect? Patients are generally thrilled with their new physique, which can only be fully appreciated with bodylift surgery following major weight loss.

What techniques do you use and why? I perform thigh, upper and lower bodylifts, and armlifts in one or more stages, depending on the needs of each patient. Sometimes the best results occur when these procedures are performed in tandem, creating a smoother contour and more skin firmness from head to toe.

Will I be bruised following the procedure and when will I see results? Although most bruising and swelling will disappear within three weeks, some swelling may remain for six months to a year. Similar to a tummy tuck, you will be able to see your new shape in four to six weeks.

How long will the procedure take? Bodylifting is major surgery, and may take three to five hours, depending on what aspects of the body are addressed.

How long does it take most of your patients to recover or return to work following bodylift? You may return to work in two to three weeks, depending on the extent of surgery.

What is the likelihood of "touch up" or "refinement" procedures? Many patients who undergo bodylifting procedures will have a second stage operation at a later date. As the scars may be unpredictable, a scar revision may be needed or liposuction for residual fat deposits.

Do you have before and after photographs of the procedure? We have in-office photographs to show you.

What Happens After Bariatric Surgery?

Bariatric or weight loss surgery reduces the size of the stomach and/or digestive tract to limit the intake of calories, or to bypass certain parts of the intestinal tract to limit absorption of calories, resulting in massive weight loss over the course of several months or years. The best candidates for bariatric surgery include those with a body mass index (BMI) above 40—approximately 100 pounds overweight for men and 80 pounds overweight for women. In some cases, people with a BMI between 35 and 40 who suffer from type II diabetes or life-threatening cardiopulmonary problems such as hypertension, severe sleep apnea, or obesity-related heart disease may also be candidates for weight loss surgery.

Following substantial weight loss, either as a result of bariatric surgery or after diet and exercise, you will typically have multiple areas of significant excess skin including the breasts, upper arms, abdomen, back, and thighs. Areas can be tightened and redundant skin can be removed in the form of a breastlift, upper armlift, tummy tuck, lower bodylift and thighlift, respectively. You may also be a candidate for facial cosmetic surgery including neck recontouring and facelifts. Due to the large amount of excess skin to be removed, usually from several different areas, it is common to require at least two or three surgical stages to achieve the best result.

BODY SHAPING STAGES

Many gastric bypass and lap-band patients seek this procedure after they have lost weight. After the weight is gone, you may be left with a lot of extra hanging skin, which may cause you to be embarrassed or self-conscious. The loose skin does not respond to diet or exercise. Only body contouring surgery will reduce the often extreme degrees of excess skin that develop with massive weight loss. Thigh, body, and armlifts all aim to "lift" and tighten the skin for a smooth appearance.

As the number of Americans having weight loss surgery increases, so does the number of individuals undergoing plastic surgery to reshape their bodies after they've lost massive amounts of weight. In 2005, more than 68,000 people underwent body contouring surgery procedures, according to the most recent statistics just released by the American Society of Plastic Surgeons. Of that number, 76 percent had undergone weight loss surgery.

Reconstructive surgery can help restore a more natural look to your body. However, in many cases, these procedures are done in stages. I will often examine patients to determine how much can be done in one procedure. A common combination might be a lower bodylift in one stage, and an armlift and breastlift in a second stage. It's important to set your priorities. The more procedures done in one stage, the more risky and the longer the recovery will be.

BODYLIFTS

For many people who lose a substantial amount of weight, the resulting rolls of loose skin seem like a poor trade off. Bodylift surgery can literally get them into bathing suit shape.

Bodylifts are ideal for people who have a significant weight loss—either from diet and exercise, or a gastric bypass procedure—who have been left with unsightly loose rolls of excess skin. It is the most effective technique to restore firm, youthful contours to the body. While exercise is an excellent way to burn calories and lose weight and to improve muscle mass and tone, it has no effect on loose, hanging skin. Lower bodylifts can address the thighs, buttocks, abdomen, waist, and hips all in one stage. The added benefits are an overall improvement in dimpling and cellulite, as well as an elevation of the pubic area to a more youthful status. Bodylifts may also be performed after previous liposuction. If there is excess skin after fat removal, a thighlift, abdominoplasty, or lower bodylift may be performed to reduce the amount of loose tissue.

The Bodylift is considered an extension of an abdominoplasty; it reduces the excess skin and fat deposits of the central body region, including abdomen, hips, thighs and buttocks.

How We Do It

Bodylift surgery is usually performed under general anesthesia because it involves a large surgical area and can be quite extensive. For thighlifts, excess skin is lifted and removed through incisions made in the inner thigh and/or high upper outer thigh. Simultaneous lifting of the thighs and buttocks is done using incisions that follow a high-cut bathing suit line only a bit higher up on the hip. We lift and remove the excess skin and fat down to the muscle. Drain tubes may be placed at the incision to draw out fluids. The lifting surgery can be combined with limited liposuction. Some of the scars can be hidden in the natural skin creases and others are located in areas normally covered by clothing.

Quick Facts: Bodylifts

- The number of patients seeking plastic surgery for body contouring after dramatic weight loss has risen by at least 20 percent (ASAPS)

- Bodylifting procedures should not be undertaken until your weight is stable

- After bariatric surgery, it may take six months to a year before you can have a bodylift

What to Expect Afterward

The recovery from a bodylift procedure is very similar to a tummy tuck. However, my patients routinely stay in the hospital for one to two nights after surgery. It is important to walk as soon as possible after surgery to reduce the chance of blood clot formation in your legs. The swelling is mild to moderate, and peaks at two to three days. Surgical drains may be placed for several days following the procedure that will have to be emptied. For the first week following surgery, you must avoid bending or lifting. Usually the incisions are covered with adhesive steri-strips and surgical gauze. Due to the location of the incisions, it may be impossible for you to avoid lying on them. Changing position at least every 30 minutes and moving around carefully will limit stress on the incision lines.

You will have several layers of stitches with bodylift procedures. Some will be resorbed by the body and some may need to be removed by your surgeon. You will usually be able to shower on the second day after surgery. Moderate pain can be anticipated after this procedure. Areas of numbness near the incisions may occur but usually disappear gradually over several months. Although most bruising and swelling will disappear within three weeks, some swelling may remain for six months or longer. After bodylifts, you cannot resume rigorous aerobic exercise like jogging or contact sports for approximately six weeks.

Potential Pitfalls

Most lifts require fairly lengthy incisions, and scarring is an important consideration. The incisions can usually be hidden under most bathing suits. In some patients, fluid can collect beneath the skin that may need to be aspirated with a needle. Bleeding, infection, and wound healing complications including delayed healing and skin loss may occur after bodylift procedures. Swelling is significant and will take several months to settle down fully.

Armlift (Brachioplasty)

Armlift or brachioplasty is performed to surgically eliminate loose, hanging skin from the upper arms. Aging, long-term excessive sun exposure, and significant weight loss can all lead to a loss of skin elasticity. We will evaluate your upper arms to assess the amount and location of the fatty tissue as well as the degree of skin laxity. In patients with relatively good skin tone, liposuction alone may be all that is recommended for contour improvement. While liposuction can be performed to reduce the amount of fatty tissue in the upper arms, there will be little if any skin tightening effect. Excess fat is generally only removed by liposuction from the inner aspect of the arm through small incisions located along the inner elbow and the posterior aspect of the armpit. If the skin is loose and has poor tone, an armlift is the only procedure that will lead to a significant contour improvement. Liposuction is commonly performed prior to brachioplasty to maximize the aesthetic result.

How We Do It

In the standing position, we mark the area of excess skin to be removed. The incision is usually placed on the inner surface of the upper arm, and may extend from the elbow to the armpit. The pattern of the tissue to be removed is designed in such a way that the resulting scar cannot be seen from the front or back view when your arms are held at your side. Of course, the scar may be visible when you raise your arms. Incisions are sometimes made on the inner and under surface of your arm in a zigzag pattern for better healing. In some cases, skin excision may be limited to the axillary or underarm area. After the excess skin and fat are removed, the remaining skin is brought together and sutured and the incisions are covered with adhesive strips. A drain may be placed prior to skin closure to eliminate excess fluid, depending on the amount of skin and fat removed. While you are still in the operating room, elastic bandages or some type of a compression garment are applied to help control swelling.

What to Expect Afterward

During the first week after the procedure, your arms should be elevated as much as possible. Some type of compression garment should be worn at all times, except when showering, for three to four weeks. We also advise waiting at least three to four weeks before engaging in aerobic exercise and six weeks for any upper arm workouts. Some tightness could remain in the area for up to three months. The scars may remain pink for up to one year.

Potential Pitfalls

Remember: Scars are unpredictable and may not be able to be prevented or may heal in an unsightly way with armlifts. The scars from an armlift are permanent and may be visible in any position other than when the arms are hanging at the sides. If you have had a mastectomy, you are advised not to have an armlift, since the surgery interrupts some of the lymphatic drainage and the combined procedures may cause the arm to swell permanently (lymphedema). If you have a history of phlebitis or inflamed blood vessels in either arm you should not undergo brachioplasty.

It is common for women to want breast and body contouring procedures after their childbearing years to address the changes in their breasts and abdomen. We frequently perform breastlifts with or without implants at the same time as a tummy tuck or liposuction. It is generally recommended to have tummy tucks and breastlifts performed after you have your last child, as future pregnancies and breast feeding may reverse some of the tightening and lifting effects of the surgery. I like my patients to be at their baseline weight post-pregnancy before having any type of cosmetic surgery.

STRAIGHT FROM THE HEART

Caroline is an executive assistant who lost 90 pounds in time for her 40th birthday.
Age: 40
Size before bariatric surgery: 14
Size after bariatric surgery: 6

"I struggled with weight as a child. My mom was overweight, and my father gave us junk food as a reward for behaving. So I grew up with some bad habits. When I got married, my husband loved it because I never minded when he invited the guys over to watch football games, and they would fill the fridge with chips, dip, wings, beer and tons of other diet no-no's. I was the cool wife who would dig right in and eat, no matter how many carbs or grams of fat. He never cared that I was a bit on the round side; he said I was beautiful and so much more fun than women who constantly fussed and primped.

"I was secure enough in myself and my marriage to know that I didn't need to lose weight for him. But the turning point for me came around my 39th birthday, when I started thinking about the milestone birthday right around the corner. I looked at the clothes hanging in my closet and realized I had nothing that wasn't elastic, spandex, button down or wrap. Basically, everything was large enough NOT to hug my body. I missed seeing the definition in my hips. I actually missed having smaller, perkier breasts.

"Without telling my husband, I embarked on a plan to drop some serious weight by the time I turned 40. I worked out with a trainer, cut down on the junk food calories, and ate tons of lean meats, fish, vegetables, and fruits. I completely gave up soda and alcohol. In a matter of months, I had already lost 30 pounds, and the weight kept coming off. I was never a big-boned girl; I was just an overeater with bad habits.

"Once I reached the target weight loss goal of 90 pounds, I had a new problem—loose skin. I still worked out daily but the skin was still hanging around. My husband was so impressed at all of my hard work, that I thought he would be supportive if I took it one step further and got rid of the excess skin once and for all. I can honestly say it was the smartest decision I ever made. There is just no way I could have toned up as much as I did without surgery. My husband was amazing, and he took a few weeks off work to make sure I was comfortable and healed. Now, I am thinner than I have ever been—thin enough to fit into a sexy bathing suit I just bought for

our trip to Aruba, where my husband and I are planning to renew our wedding vows."

CHECKLIST

- [ ] If you lose 80 to100 pounds but have excess skin, bariatric surgery is ideal for you
- [ ] Breast and body work make a perfect pair
- [ ] Incisions can be hidden but some scarring is to be expected

CHAPTER 6

Mostly For Men

Where the Boys Are

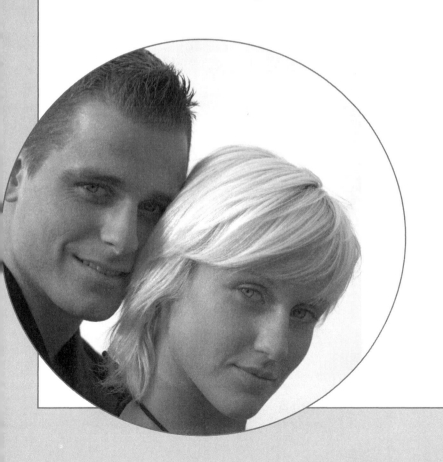

What's Hot
- A great head of hair
- Looking good for your age or younger
- Taking control of the way you look and feel

What's Not
- The stigma that cosmetic surgery is only for women
- A haphazard approach to grooming
- Missing out on the advances of modern technology

You may have never look like Brad Pitt (or have the good fortune to date a woman who looks like Angelina Jolie), but that does not mean you can't indulge in some of the image enhancing techniques available exclusively to men. This chapter is devoted exclusively to the issues men face when considering cosmetic surgery. While the numbers are still lagging behind, a notable percentage of men are seeking cosmetic surgery to improve their looks and their confidence. According to the American Society for Aesthetic Plastic Surgery, men account for nine percent of the total procedures performed.

TOP 5 MALE PROCEDURES (ASAPS)

1. Liposuction

2. Rhinoplasty

3. Blepharoplasty

4. Male Breast Reduction

5. Facelift

GREENBERG'S LIST
Top 5 Male Reasons for Avoiding Cosmetic Enhancements

1. My dad had thinning hair, I have thinning hair—it's just a fact of life

2. I don't have time to take off work to have cosmetic surgery

3. I'm not that vain—only women get surgery

4. I'm working with a trainer to get rid of that bulge

5. I don't want my friends to know that I had anything done

In my practice, men constitute about 30 percent of my patients. Their wives and girlfriends often bring them in, but many men come in on their own for injectables as well as surgery.

THINNING HAIR

As we age, the rate of hair growth slows. The most common cause of thinning hair is heredity and can be passed down from either your mother's or your father's side of the family. You may notice areas of hair that no longer need cutting, and where the hairs are getting shorter and finer. It is important to know that finding hairs in your tub, sink, or brush is not necessarily a sign of thinning hair. This could indicate a temporary hair loss condition. It is natural for hair to go through a constant cycle of growth and resting or dormancy. If you are not on your way to balding, your hair will grow back just as strong. If you are balding, your hair will grow back finer, and will not grow as long before falling out again. What you see in the mirror over a longer period is the best monitor of early signs of thinning.

Hair Loss Drugs

The main drugs that are approved by the FDA for treatment of hair loss are:

Minoxidil (Rogaine®) This over-the-counter medication is approved for the treatment of androgenetic alopecia and alopecia areata. Minoxidil is a liquid that you rub into your scalp twice daily to regrow hair and to prevent further loss. Minoxidil is available in a two percent solution and in a five percent solution. New hair resulting from minoxidil use may be thinner and shorter than previous hair. But there can be enough regrowth for some people to hide their bald spots and have it blend with existing hair. Side effects can include scalp irritation. New hair stops growing soon after you discontinue the use of minoxidil.

Finasteride (Propecia®, Proscar®) This prescription medication to treat male-pattern baldness is taken daily in pill form. Many men taking finasteride experience a slowing of hair loss, and some may show some new hair growth. Positive results may take several months. Finasteride works by inhibiting the conversion of testosterone into dihydrotestosterone (DHT), a hormone that shrinks hair follicles and is an important factor in male hair loss. Rare side effects include a diminished sex drive. As with minoxidil, the benefits stop if usage is discontinued.

New Hair Transplant Techniques

Improved surgical techniques can achieve better hair follicle survival, take less time to perform, and leave fewer scars at the back and sides of the head. Transplanted hair is removed from one area (donor site) and transferred to another (recipient site). The newly transplanted hair maintains its color and texture, and grows naturally. Many years ago, large circular grafts called 'hair plugs' containing 15 to 20 hairs were transplanted resulting in very obvious, often embarrassing results.

We have found that hair grows from the scalp in groups of one to four follicular units. We can transfer these follicles to be placed closer together to create a dense looking head of hair. In most hair transplant procedures, healthy hair follicles are excised surgically from the back of the head where hair growth is permanent and thicker. An aesthetically pleasing, thin scar at the donor site after multiple hair-restoration procedures is the ultimate goal.

Transplanting groups of hair follicles has improved the cosmetic results of hair restoration and made the procedure shorter. We can now recreate hairlines and crown coverage that looks totally natural, unlike the old techniques that looked very obvious. It is important to have an understanding for the natural patterns of hair growth to get a good aesthetic result.

Quick Facts: Hair Loss

- The most common cause of hair loss is heredity

- Men are most commonly affected by the inherited gene

- 35 million men in the US are losing their hair (ISHRS)

- Hair loss in men occur most frequently between from late teens to the 40s and 50s

The Chest Wall

Affecting almost 40 percent of men, gynecomastia is the enlargement of the male breast. The male breast appears fuller and rounded compared with the ideal flattened and rectangular male breast contour. Typically, gynecomastia is caused by a combination of dense breast tissue behind the nipple and fatty tissue over the pectoralis major muscle. The fullness of the male breast is detected by firmness just below the nipple, extends around the side to the edge of the pectoralis muscle and into the armpits. True gynecomastia is a proliferation of the glandular breast tissue with or without increased fat accumulation. Most often, men want a flatter, more defined breast and chest shape as well as flatter and smaller nipples and areola (the pigmented area of the nipple). Men may be embarrassed and feel extremely self-conscious about their feminized appearing chest.

In order to determine the appropriate treatment, I have to examine the breast thoroughly to determine the prominent tissue types and to evaluate the size of the breast enlargement. Surgery to reduce the size of the male breast can be done in an outpatient surgical facility. Local or general anesthesia is used. Aggressive liposuction alone may be sufficient in some cases. I use traditional tumescent liposuction with specialized cannulae for this procedure. In some cases, ultrasonic assisted liposuction (UAL) helps to dissolve the fibrous fat and produces a better result.

In cases where liposuction alone is not effective, minimal incision surgery is used to remove the firm breast tissue through an incision that is hidden at the edge of the areola. The areolar approach demonstrates a more cosmetically pleasing result since the scar does not extend to the surrounding skin. Occasionally a patient has an abundance of extra skin. We first remove the fat and breast tissue and wait about a year for the skin to retract. If the skin remains, we may have to remove it in a year.

After surgery, you will wear a light compression garment, worn for several weeks as a dressing. Recovery is often uncomplicated. You can resume normal activities within days, and even shower two days after surgery. Peaking at two to three days, swelling is mild to moderate and disappears rapidly over the next three weeks. Minimal or no bruising is normal. Dissolving sutures are placed under the skin so there are no sutures to remove. After swelling disappears, expect a permanent, balanced, and proportioned contour. There will be some firmness in all the treated areas that takes several months to resolve.

Pectoral Implants

Male chest enhancement is growing in popularity as more men are choosing to enhance their physiques, body symmetry, and self-image with pectoral implants. Pec implants give a more prominent and muscular appearing chest and correct unevenness from one side to the other. This procedure can enhance an already toned physique for men who just cannot achieve the chest size that they desire through weight lifting alone. Pec implants may also be used to simulate the effects of spending hours at the gym. It can be combined with reducing the size of the nipples and areolae as well.

Pectoral augmentation involves inserting a soft, high grade, solid silicone implant into a space created under the pectoral muscles. To the touch, it will have the consistency of a flexed muscle. Unlike female breast augmentation, after this procedure is properly completed and healed, you will probably not require additional surgery in the future. Frequently, liposuction of the love handles, abdomen, and waist is performed to further enhance the overall shape and contour of the torso.

Pec implants are made of soft silicone block. They cannot leak or spread since there is no gel or fluid. They come in different shapes and sizes to accommodate any anatomic features and the cosmetic look you desire. Generally, scars are easily hidden in the armpit area within the hair bearing skin so they are not visible.

How We Do It

This procedure is usually performed on an outpatient basis under general or local anesthesia with intravenous sedation. The surgery takes approximately one to two hours. An incision is made high in your armpit, about two inches long, that is used to create a space between the two chest wall muscles—the pectoralis major and the pectoralis minor. The implant is placed between these two muscles. It is well camouflaged and safe in this position. A "pocket" or space is created under each pectoral muscle of the chest corresponding to the planned outline on the skin, which was marked prior to surgery. The solid silicone pectoral implants are then inserted. The incision is closed with sutures below the level of the skin to avoid cross-hatching and suture marks. At the conclusion of surgery a light dressing and elastic compression garment is applied over the surgical area. These are worn for about three to four weeks or less.

What to Expect Afterward

Following the surgery, you may experience mild to moderate pain which is easily controlled with medication and rapidly subsides after two days. Varying degrees of swelling and bruising peak at two to three days and then subside over several weeks. Gentle arm raising maneuvers may be resumed immediately after surgery. You can shower and wash in two days. The elastic compression garment or bandage is generally worn for one to two weeks following surgery. You may return to your routine activities after two weeks, and start doing lower body exercises in two to three weeks. Full workouts are permitted after four to six weeks. The results usually look very natural, even when flexing or working your muscles, and that does not change or sag over time.

Potential Pitfalls

Possible complications include: anesthesia risks, bleeding, infection, fluid accumulation under the skin (seroma), which may need to be drained, nerve damage, poor wound healing, and unsatisfactory scars. Asymmetry, displacement, or hardening of the scar tissue around the implant, and the need for removal of the implants may occur.

Body Sculpting via Liposuction

As a man gains weight, his fat cells expand. As he loses weight, the fat cells contract in size, but the number and distribution remain essentially unchanged. Dieting reduces your weight and overall size, and may show improvement in specific areas. Liposuction, on the other hand, reduces the total number of fat cells and therefore, affects shape and contour, so future weight gain or loss will not be noticed as much in the areas that were treated. It is a safe and effective way to remove bulges to produce an improved shape and contour.

Most areas of your body can be suctioned, from the face down to the ankles. Stubborn fat deposits that do not respond to exercise and diet regimens are ideal targets for liposuction. Men tend to accumulate fat deposits in the midsection—typically the abdomen, waist, and chest. In some cases, fat deposits may also show up in the thigh area in men. Several areas are frequently combined in one stage to maximize the potential for the skin to shrink after the fat is removed. However, the typical "beer belly" with fat located within the abdominal cavity, cannot be suctioned at all.

> *Liposuction is ideal for removing fatty breast tissue and giving men back the abs they had in college.*

Liposuction can remove love handles that even gym rats can't shed through vigorous training. Results from liposuction will be best if you continue regular workouts at the gym after the procedure. Men often have more resilient skin than women, so it tends to shrink better following the procedure.

Top Areas for Male Liposuction

1. Flanks (love handles)

2. Abdomen

3. Chest

4. Chin

Male Tummy Tucks

There is a wide variation in the procedures I perform on men for the torso. The most common is liposuction alone, and the more invasive is a panniculectomy, which involves removing an apron of skin and fat, or a bodylift. Men are also candidates for abdominoplasty, where I transpose the umbilicus and tighten the muscles of the abdominal wall. It is much more common for men to have abdominoplasty. Men can typically go back to work in about two weeks.

Age-Defying Procedures That Really Work

Courtesy of

Stephen T. Greenberg, MD, FACS
OBAGI® MEDICAL PRODUCTS
Q-MED
SYNERON MEDICAL

FACELIFT & BLEPHROPLASTY

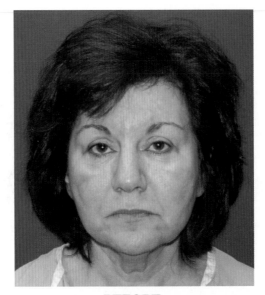

BEFORE

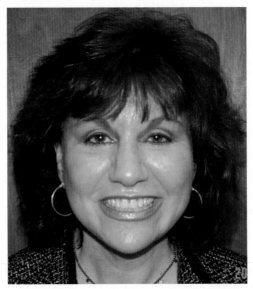

AFTER

FACELIFT & BLEPHROPLASTY

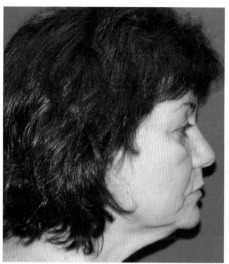

BEFORE

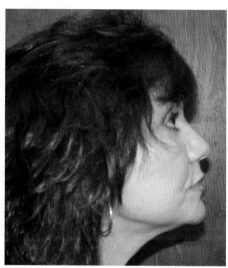

AFTER

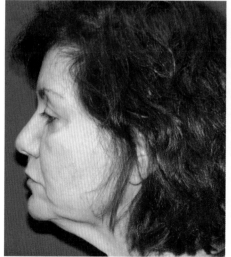

BEFORE

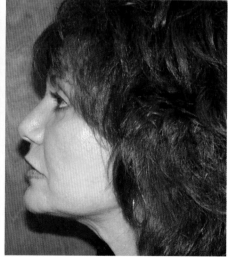

AFTER

RESTYLANE®

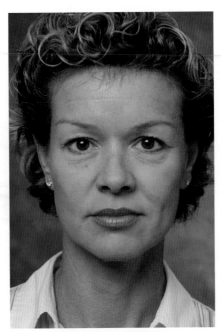

BEFORE—FRONT

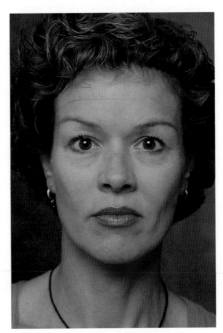

AFTER—FRONT

Restylane® in lips, oral commisures and nasolabial folds.

RESTYLANE®

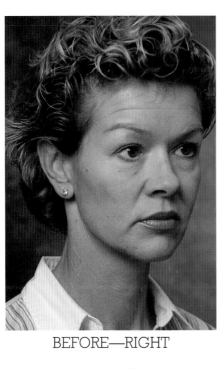

BEFORE—RIGHT

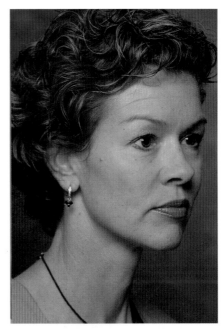

AFTER—RIGHT

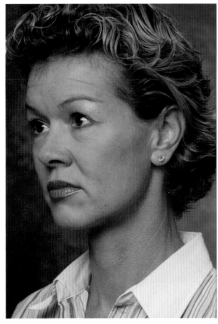

BEFORE—LEFT

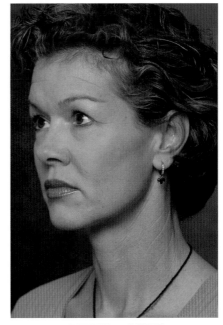

AFTER—LEFT

Restylane® in lips, oral commisures and nasolabial folds.

RHINOPLASTY

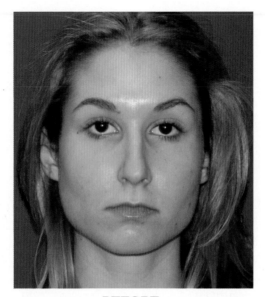

BEFORE

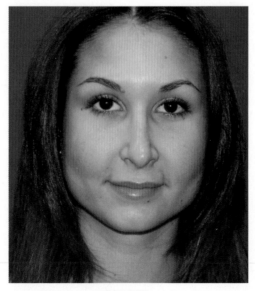

AFTER

RHINOPLASTY

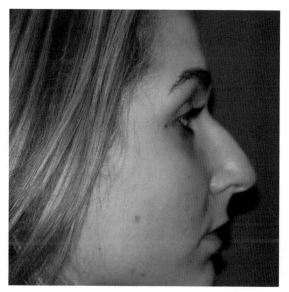

BEFORE

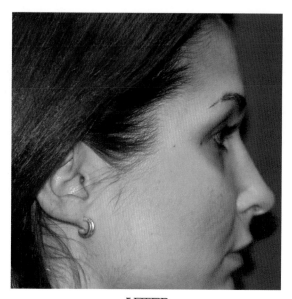

AFTER

LIPOSUCTION

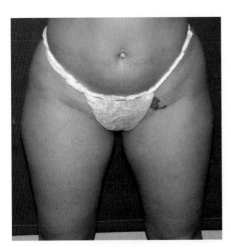

BEFORE

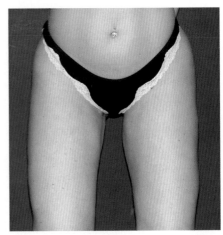

AFTER

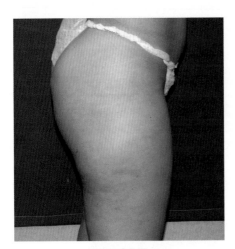

BEFORE

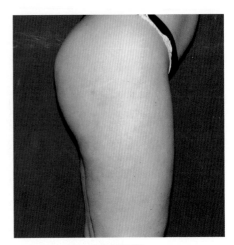

AFTER

TUMMY TUCK

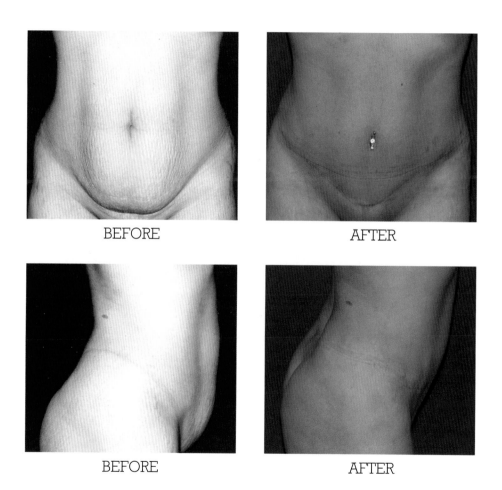

BEFORE AFTER

BEFORE AFTER

BREAST LIFT & AUGMENTATION

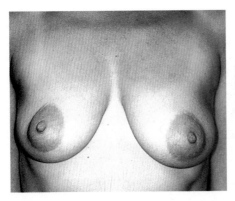

BEFORE

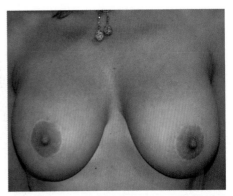

AFTER

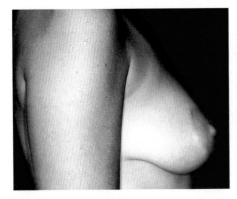

BEFORE

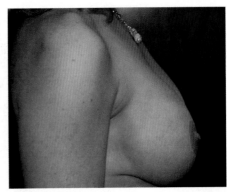

AFTER

BREAST AUGMENTATION

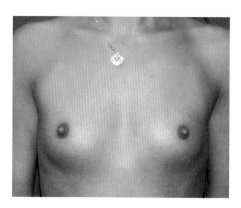

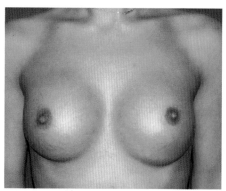

BEFORE

AFTER

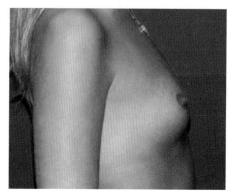

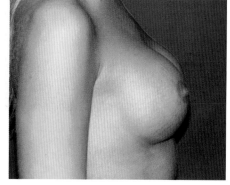

BEFORE

AFTER

REFIRME™
SYNERON MEDICAL

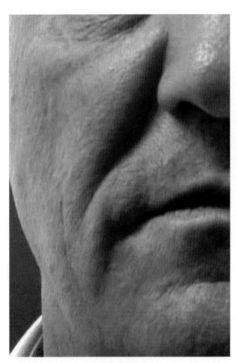 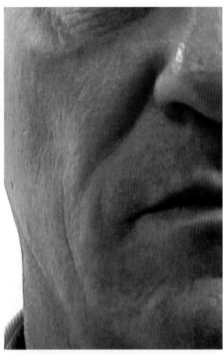

BEFORE   AFTER

OBAGI®

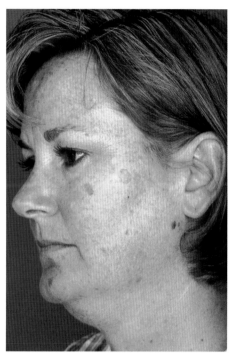

BEFORE

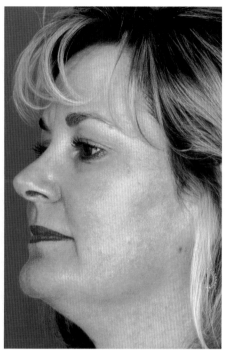

AFTER

Duration of Treatment: 12 weeks
Treatment Protocol: Obagi Nu-Derm System and 1 Obagi Blue Peel

OBAGI®

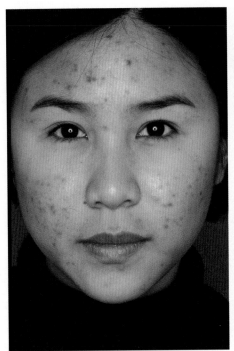 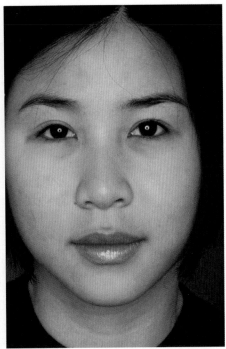

BEFORE   AFTER

Treatment Protocol: Obagi Nu-Derm System
Duration of Treatment: 14 week

OBAGI®

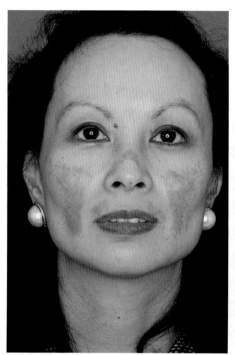

BEFORE

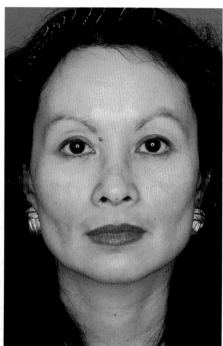

AFTER

Treatment Protocol: Obagi Nu-Derm System
Duration of Treatment: 18 weeks

Stephen T. Greenberg, MD
Proudly Announces
The Introduction of his

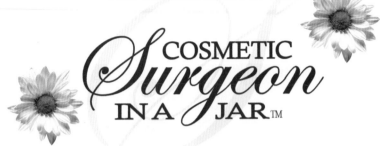

COSMETIC Surgeon IN A JAR™

Anti-aging Formula Skin Care System.
Each product in this anti-aging
skin care system contains a combination
of both the newest and most established
proven ingredients, that were personally
selected and tested by
Dr. Greenberg and his product advisory team.

The 6 synergistic products are:
TRIPLE ACTION EYE SERUM
BRIGHTENING COMPLEXION CREAM
FIRMING & TIGHTENING CREAM
ULTIMATE SKIN EXFOLIATOR
REVITALIZING pH BALANCED TONER
ANTIOXIDANT CLEANSING FOAM

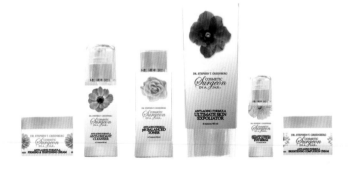

For more information visit Dr. Greenberg's Web site:
www.greenbergcosmeticsurgery.com
www.alittlenipalittletuck.com

Buttock Recontouring

This procedure that has become more popular in men who desire
a more youthful appearance of the buttock region. This may involve
enlargement, reduction, or lift. Sagging and flabby buttocks related
to aging, weight loss, or produced by too much liposuction can be
improved. To enlarge the buttocks, the most common procedure is fat
grafting, which produces a higher, rounder buttocks. It also lifts sagging
buttocks to some degree. Fat is injected into
the gluteus muscle and into the fat spaces.
Silicone buttock implants can also be placed
beneath the muscle through a four-inch
incision. Dressings and a light compression
garment are worn for several weeks, but
there are no stitches to remove. Expect some
discomfort that is easily tolerated by the second or third day, and may be controlled with
pain medications. Peaking at two to three
days, swelling is mild to moderate and then
disappears rapidly over the next three weeks.
Minimal bruising is normal. Some grogginess
will persist for several days. You can shower
on the second day after surgery. You can resume many activities within
the first week, and most by at least three weeks post-surgery. You can
expect to be out of work for three to seven days. The best way to contour the buttocks is through liposuction.

Greenberg's Guys Who Look Great:

- Matthew McConaughey
- George Clooney
- Jude Law
- Clive Owen
- Orlando Bloom
- Taye Diggs
- Brad Pitt
- Ashton Kutcher

STRAIGHT FROM THE HEART

**Keith is a successful investment banker on Wall Street looking
for a an upgrade.**
Age: 35
Height: 6'1
Weight: 198

"I really thought cosmetic surgery was the last thing I would ever

do. I'm pretty active even though my job is very demanding and the hours can be grueling. I just made time to go for a run every morning or even sometimes late at night. It got to the point where the runs just were not cutting it anymore. Even intense workouts were not getting rid of the gut that was slowly growing around my midsection. I thought about seeing a cosmetic surgeon for a few months, and every time I reached for the phone, I just couldn't psych myself up to take that first step. I kept imagining my Marine father calling me a wimp who didn't know the first thing about getting in shape.

"It took some time and a lot of research for me to realize that a lot of men were actually doing things to improve their looks and their bodies. The truth is, we expect women to look flawless, but most people don't look that way naturally. The shame factor was a big hurdle for me to overcome, but I finally set up a consultation, and Dr. Greenberg suggested liposuction. I laughed because I used to think that was something only women in movies who lived in Beverly Hills did every few years.

"Going in for surgery was kind of a rush. I talked everything over with Dr. Greenberg, looked at pictures, and we discussed potential problems that could arise, so I knew the kind of result I was going to get. I took about ten days off from work—I travel a fair amount for business so no one even knew why I was gone. When I got back to the office, I got a lot of positive feedback. My female colleagues commented that my suits hung well on me, or asked me how I lost the weight. It feels amazing to have this kind of result—it's a huge confidence boost!"

CHECKLIST

- [ ] Men: there is no shame in cosmetic surgery—men, you deserve to look good too!
- [ ] No need to accept thinning hair without a fight!
- [ ] From chest sculpting to buttock augmentation, there's more than one way to tone and tighten your body

CHAPTER 7

The Eyes Have It!

The Windows to the Soul

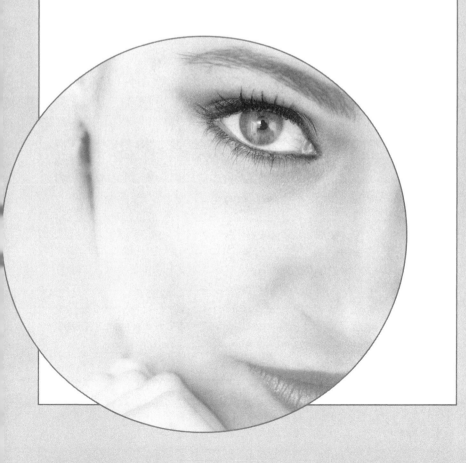

What's Hot
- A brilliant pair of eyes to set of a gorgeous face
- A wide eyed, open, fresh appearance
- A smooth brow that begs the question, "Does she or doesn't she?"

What's Not
- The "deer in the headlights" look
- Cat eyes
- Bags that add ten years

Your eyes are a focal point of your face and give others clues about your age, mood, and whether you are tired or well rested. When beginning the process of facial rejuvenation, many people choose eyelid surgery as a starting point. One of the main reasons may be that your eyelids often show the effects of aging, gravity, sun exposure, and smoking before the rest of your face or neck.

The first impression is the one most remembered—so you should always put your best face forward. You may have flawless skin, full lips and great cheekbones, but tired, droopy eyes can be seen a mile away. Fortunately, there are a wide range of procedures that will play up your sparklers and give you a more beautiful face in the process.

GREENBERG'S LIST
Top Questions for Your Eye and Brow Surgery

How long have you been doing eye surgery procedures? At least three years is preferable.

How many eye and brow procedures do you perform each week? At least three to five is preferable.

What kind of results can I expect? A more open look, contoured brows, and smoother lower eyelid and upper cheek region.

What techniques do you use and why? I perform lower and upper eyelid surgery and fat removal using techniques that provide well-hidden, minimal scarring. I often combine an eyelift with a browlift, which creates a younger looking upper face.

How long will the procedure take? About an hour.

***Will I be bruised following the procedure and when will I see
results?*** Some swelling and bruising is to be expected for one week in most cases.

***How long does it take most of your patients to recover or return to
work following an eyelift or browlift?*** You can resume activities like read-
ing and using a computer the following day, but on a limited basis. Most patients can
return to work quickly, in one week.

What is the likelihood of "touch up" or "refinement" procedures?
While the procedure may need to be revised at some point in the future if there is very
loose or thin skin, effects generally last ten years or more.

EYELID LIFT (UPPER/LOWER BLEPHAROPLASTY)

Women and men with baggy under-eyes or droopy upper eyelids will
notice a great improvement in their appearance with eyelid surgery.
Much of what happens to the skin around our eyes as we age is heredi-
tary. Even if you cannot fight your genes, you can stave off the effects
of time with rejuvenating eyelid surgery.

Protruding fatty tissue from your eye sockets that causes bulging
above or below the eye can be an inherited trait that shows up early
in life, but it can also be the result of aging. Generalized sun exposure
over the years will have a direct effect on the weakening of your
elastic fibers that keep eyelid skin taut. Eyelid skin and muscle thin and
stretch with time. Bulging fat pockets result when fat pads that cushion
the eyes begin to fall forward, pull away from the bone of the lower
eyelids, and sag.

Aging upper eyelids may cause a hood to form over the eyelashes
where your upper lids have become heavier and fuller. Blepharoplasty
can get rid of droopy or hooded eyelids and eliminate the protruding
fat bags above and below your eyes. In some cases, cosmetic eyelid
surgery may be combined with surgery to correct a functional problem
such as weakness of upper eyelid muscles called "ptosis" (pronounced
toe-sis) that can decrease the range of upward vision.

The goal of eyelid rejuvenation techniques is to remove excess skin,
reduce fat deposits or reposition them, to tighten lax eyelid muscles,
and to re-establish a natural crease in the upper lids. We preserve the

fat whenever possible to avoid creating an operated look or cause hollows around your eyes. The effects generally last ten years or more, and leave you looking fresh and rejuvenated. Often, the procedure does not even need to be repeated.

How We Do It

Excess fat, skin, and, if needed, muscle are removed from your upper and/or lower eyelids. The procedure is performed on an outpatient basis under local anesthesia with intravenous sedation or under general anesthesia, especially when it is combined with another surgical procedure. First, eye drops may be used to anesthetize your eyes, and then an ointment may be placed in your eyes to protect the globes during the surgery. We use very fine electrocautery throughout eyelid surgery to minimize bleeding.

Dr. Greenberg's Most Requested Enviable Eyes

- Catherine Zeta-Jones
- Mariska Hargitay
- Penelope Cruz
- Adriana Lima
- Liz Hurley
- Kimora Lee Simmons

Lower Eyelids

The most common methods of performing lower blepharoplasty are the external approach—also called a skin-muscle flap—and the transconjunctival approach. For the external approach, the incision begins at a point near the inner tear duct of the lower eyelid, approximately two to three millimeters below the eyelash line, and typically extends into the crow's feet area where lines already exist so that the scar will be less noticeable. We lift the skin and muscle to remove a small amount of fat. Excess skin and muscle are then trimmed from the lower lid.

If you have a pocket of fat beneath your lower eyelids but do not have any loose skin, we may recommend a transconjunctival blepharoplasty. It is usually performed on younger people with fatty lower eyelids and taut skin. The transconjunctival method utilizes an incision hidden inside the lower eyelid which leaves no visible external scars.

Through this incision, the surgeon exposes and trims the excess fat. The incision is closed with dissolving sutures or, more commonly, it is left to heal on its own.

A lower eyelid tightening procedure may also be performed with an eyelid lift using either surgical approach, but if significant skin and muscle laxity are present, the skin muscle flap (external) approach is advisable.

Another aspect of lower eyelid surgery addresses the "tear troughs" or deep grooves that can result when there is an obvious demarcation at the junction of the lower eyelid area and the cheek. The main methods for improving the tear trough area are fat removal, fat injections, or fat transposition to move around the existing fatty deposits to create a smoother look.

These depressions are often difficult to treat. Some patients have a "pouch" that sits lower than the lower eyelid. These are called malar fat pads and do not go away with lower eyelid surgery.

Upper Eyelids

Upper blepharoplasty involves making an elliptical incision across the eyelid crease, in the natural skin fold. We draw a line to identify the lower edge of the skin to be excised, which will eventually become the scar that remains. The loose and redundant skin of your upper eyelid is then marked out. Excess skin and fatty tissue are removed along with a thin strip of muscle to give your eyelid crease more definition. We close the incision with a single layer of fine sutures. When correctly planned, the scar is well hidden within the natural fold of your upper eyelids.

What to Expect Afterward

Thin surgical tape is sometimes applied to your stitch line after the surgery. An ointment to prevent dryness may be applied but it is not necessary for your eyes to be covered. Your eyelids will feel tight and sore as the anesthesia wears off and you may feel a slight burning sensation along the suture lines. Although you will be able to read, use a computer and watch television the next day, these activities should be limited because they tend to dry the eyes and your eyes will tire easily. Head elevation with extra pillows above the level of the heart is important when you are lying down to help minimize swelling. Applying cold compresses or ice packs for the first 48 hours will also help to reduce your swelling. Some swelling and bruising is to be expected for several weeks, depending on the extent of your procedure.

The stitches are removed three to five days after the procedure. For seven to ten days, the eye area will need to be cleaned and your eyes may feel sticky and itchy. In some cases, we recommend using artificial tears for lubrication that will help the gritty or scratchy feeling in the first few days after surgery.

You should not wear contact lenses for one week and you may feel uncomfortable for a while when you resume wearing them. We recommend wearing sunglasses in the first few weeks after surgery since your eyes will be sensitive to sun, wind and other irritants. For the first two weeks, avoid any activity that increases blood flow to the eyes or surrounding area including bending, lifting, crying and exercise or sports. Although your scars can remain slightly pink for six months after surgery, they should eventually fade to a thin, barely visible white line.

Potential Pitfalls

A dry eye condition or blepharitis can inhibit healing and possibly result in injury or infection of the cornea. In mild cases of dry eyes, a more conservative surgical approach is generally better. Minor adverse effects may include temporary double or blurred vision, burning, stinging, gritty sensation in the eye, excessive tearing and a slight asymmetry. Severe complications may include decreased sensation in the eyelid, dry eyes, difficulty closing your eyes completely, or an ectropion where the lower lid is pulled down. A more serious but extremely rare complication is bleeding behind the eye, called retrobulbar hematoma.

When you think you are looking tired, it may be sagging upper lids or your brows that are drooping.

BROWLIFT

As you get older, deep creases across your forehead and between your eyebrows develop and may be visible even when you are not actively raising your eyebrows or squeezing them together. And there is also a gradual descent of your normal brow position that gives your eyebrows a "heavy" look. Ideally, the eyebrow sits above the bony rim around your eye. If you place your finger on your eyebrow and it sits below the bony rim, you may consider having your brow lifted.

A browlift helps to reverse these aging changes by tightening a sagging forehead, removing and softening some creases, and lifting falling eyebrows. Younger patients should also consider this procedure if you have inherited traits such as low eyebrow position or deep frown lines. To temporarily halt wrinkles, botulinum toxin injections will treat the forehead area and between your eyebrows, and you can also plump up the deepest creases between your eyebrows with soft tissue fillers.

Browlifts are commonly performed in conjunction with facelifts or eyelid surgery. When performed in the same operative session as an upper eyelid lift, the browlift should be performed first as it will tend to minimize the amount of upper eyelid skin that needs to be removed.

There are two basic techniques that we use for lifting the brow: the older, more traditional coronal browlift and the more commonly used endoscopic browlift. We prefer the endoscopic technique for a browlift because the scalp incisions are minimized, there is a lower chance of permanent scalp numbness, and the recovery is shorter. This technique is also recommended for people with thinning hair. As with all surgery, there are many ways to achieve the same goals. We tailor our technique to your particular needs and aesthetic preferences.

A newer technique is called a thread browlift. It can be used in certain patients without the need for extensive surgery or incisions.

How We Do It

Typically, a browlift can be performed under local anesthesia with intravenous sedative to make you drowsy, or with general anesthesia.

Coronal Lift

With the coronal technique, the cut is made through your scalp slightly behind your natural hairline which runs from ear to ear across the top of your head, in the location where a headband or headset would sit. For people with a high hairline, this incision can be made where the hairline begins to avoid moving the hairline back any further. After making the incision, your scalp and forehead skin is lifted away from the underlying tissue and pulled tight, causing elevation of the eyebrows. The excess scalp tissue is trimmed away and then the incision is closed with stitches or staples. I rarely use this technique anymore because there are many less invasive alternatives that patients prefer.

Endoscopic Browlift

The endoscope, a system of special surgical instruments, allows us to work under your skin down to the internal structures. In plastic surgery, the endoscope can be very handy because the tiny viewing scope and the fine instruments that we use to do the actual work are inserted through very small, "keyhole" incisions. This results in barely noticeable scars. Instead of one long incision, the endoscopic technique requires three to five one-inch incisions and is my technique of choice. To see the underlying muscles and tissues, we insert an endoscope (a wand with a small camera on the end) into one of the incisions. In another incision, we insert a different instrument to lift the skin and release the underlying muscles and tissues. Next the eyebrows are lifted and secured underneath the skin.

We have incorporated the Endotine™ device (Coapt Systems) into our browlift procedures for added fixation. The operation results in a smooth forehead and more youthful looking eyes. This technique is also good for women who have a high hairline and don't want to move it back further, and for men who have thinning hair and do not want more invasive procedures that leave visible scars.

Temporal Lift

By making a limited incision just behind the natural hairline in the area of the temple, the outer part of your eyebrows can be elevated. This technique is mainly intended for people with slight droopiness on the outer aspects of their eyebrows who do not have a general overall lower position of their eyebrows.

ContourLift™

We can also place two to three barbed sutures on each side as another way of lifting the outer part of your eyebrows. We make small incisions along a natural forehead crease or behind your frontal hairline. Although this is a much simpler approach than an endoscopic browlift, the results are not always as long lasting.

What to Expect Afterward

To reduce swelling, you will need to keep your head elevated. Bandages are removed within a few days and stitches or staples are removed within a week. Within one to two days you can shower and shampoo your hair. Numbness, tightness of the forehead and temporary pulling around the stitch line are common. Your cheeks and eyes may also swell and bruise, but these effects should resolve within a week or so. Most people are up and about in a few days, but you should rest for at least the first week after surgery. Rigorous physical activity should be avoided for several weeks. Most of the visible signs of surgery should fade within the first two to three weeks.

Potential Pitfalls

There is a possibility that the nerves that control eyebrow movement may be injured on one or both sides, which may result in an inability to raise your eyebrows or wrinkle your forehead. This is usually a temporary condition, but may be long term or permanent in rare cases. You may have a loss of sensation along or just beyond the incision line. This is common, especially with the coronal type of browlift. Scalp numbness is usually temporary and usually resolves in six months, but may be permanent in some people. Another possible adverse consequence is the formation of a widened scar after the coronal type lift, which may require another surgical procedure to create a new, thinner scar. You may also experience hair loss or thinning hair in the vicinity of the scar, if it has been placed in the hairline. Hair growth should resume within a few weeks or months. A small degree of unevenness in eyebrow position may occur, and despite all efforts, may remain after surgery.

STRAIGHT FROM THE HEART

Lucy is a 56-year-old retired nurse with the skin of a 40 year old, looking to give her eye area a little boost.

"My mother used to frown a lot, and I remember as a child asking her why she had so many lines on her forehead and between her eyebrows. When I hit 40, I started to notice the same lines creeping up on me. I immediately called my mother and demanded that she tell me the name of every product she had ever used to combat lines and wrinkles.

"I started with Botox® and had some great results between my brows for awhile. But then I began to feel really self-conscious every time I caught a glimpse of myself in a mirror. My creases were still there. Dr. Greenberg explained that a lot of this had to do with genetics and was not something I could control on my own. He suggested a browlift to smooth out the wrinkles.

"At first I was not thrilled at the thought of surgery. It was actually my mother who ended up convincing me that I should take the plunge. She said, 'If I were your age and had your skin, I would not think twice.' I took what she said to heart, because people were

always commenting on how porcelain-like my skin was. It seemed like a shame not to do something if I could. It was getting to the point where my skin looked great, but my forehead was old.

"When I went in for surgery I was really nervous, and even though Dr. Greenberg assured me that the recovery would be easy, I prepared myself for the worst. I think going there with that attitude was probably silly, considering I had really done my homework, chosen a doctor I trusted, and knew just what to expect. But what can I say—I am a born worrier. Thankfully, it was much easier than I expected. I was in bed for a weekend, and my mother stayed with me to make sure I was well taken care of. The truth is, having her nearby was great because she encouraged me and made me feel better about my choice. I knew that I would be much happier and feel all the more attractive when it was all over. I am so glad I did it. I truly feel like I look 10 years younger."

CHECKLIST

- ☐ Genetics contributes to having a droopy brow or frown lines
- ☐ If traditional surgery is not for you, consider the less invasive ContourLift™ technique
- ☐ Eyelid rejuvenation can take 10 to15 years off your age.

DR. GREENBERG'S AFTER CARE

Elevate head as much as possible for 48 hours.

Sleep on two pillows for three to four days

Take your pain medications as prescribed; one to two by mouth every three to four hours as needed for pain

Take antibiotics by mouth until finished.

Use eye drops for four days as prescribed. Tobradex® two drops each eye three times per day. Starting day of surgery, and Refresh Tears® (Natural Tears) Day & Night (Gel)

Do not take aspirin or other anti-inflammatories for at least one week.

Do not take any vitamins for at least one week

No heavy lifting, working out or strenuous activity for at least three weeks

CONTINUED

Keep cool compresses on your eyes for 48 hours; 20 minutes on, followed by 30 minutes off.

Apply gentle pressure onto eyes for any oozing or trickling of blood.

No smoking or alcohol for 48 hours.

No driving while taking pain medications.

Eat light food for 24 hours.

Use bacitracin ophthalmic ointment on the incisions for 48 hours. This may cause slight blurry vision if it gets in your eyes. Do not use ointment on day of post-op visit.

If you have any severe change in vision, double vision, blindness, rapid swelling or other sudden changes, call your surgeon immediately.

CHAPTER 8

The Perfect Profile

The Art of Rhinoplasty

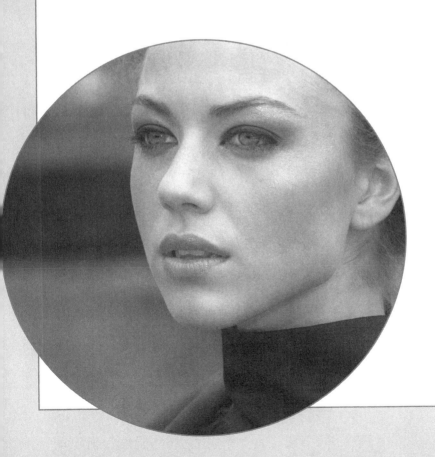

What's Hot
* Having your nose refined as an adult—not only in high school
* Preserving the character in your nose
* A nose that suits your face and does not overpower your features

What's Not
* Ski slope profiles
* Nostrils so pulled back that you can see inside your nose
* Having your nose look good, but not being able to breathe right

Never underestimate the importance of a good nose. It sits prominently in the middle of your face, so there is no way to hide that bump or that wide bridge. I see men, women, and often parents with teenagers, who have dealt with the shame and ridicule that society imposes on a less than perfect profile. It's no surprise that rhinoplasty is the most popular procedures in the U.S. among teenagers. At an age where image is everything, a nose refinement can do wonders to boost a teen's self-esteem and confidence.

GREENBERG'S LIST
Top Questions for Your Rhinoplasty

How long have you been doing rhinoplasty procedures? At least five years is preferable; rhinoplasty is one of the most difficult surgeries to master.

How many rhinoplasty procedures do you perform each week? At least three is preferable.

What kind of results can I expect? A natural looking result, an improved profile in most cases, and a nose that is in proportion with your other features, chin and upper lip contours.

What techniques do you use and why? I use both the closed and open techniques depending on what is best for each individual patient. Most patients prefer a closed technique that leaves no visible scar, whenever possible.

How long will the procedure take? One and a half hours is usually sufficient.

Will I be bruised following the procedure and when will I see results? If I break your nasal bones, you may have some bruising around your eyes. If just tip refinement is performed, you may just be swollen and have little or no bruising at all.

How long does it take most of your patients to recover or return to work following rhinoplasty? Most people can return to work, school, and to sports in four weeks.

What is the likelihood of "touch up" or "refinement" procedures? As rhinoplasty is a difficult procedure, there are cases where a secondary minor procedure may be needed to shave some cartilage or adjust the tip proportions, but this is not common.

NOSE RESHAPING (RHINOPLASTY)

The most common complaints people have regarding the appearance of their nose include large size, crookedness, a nasal hump, a wide bridge, a droopy or ill-defined thick tip and excessively flared nostrils. Noses may need to be lengthened, augmented, or narrowed for the best aesthetic result. Rhinoplasty can be used to correct a variety of conditions including the appearance of the nose and whether it is in proportion to the other facial features, as well as functional problems including nasal airway obstruction and traumatic injuries. Breathing problems related to the internal nasal structures can be corrected simultaneously with nose reshaping procedures.

Some people inherit the shape and size of their nose. In some cases, the nasal shape is a result of trauma, injury, and aging.

When I evaluate your nose, I study both the frontal view and the profile, in addition to taking note of the shape and projection of your chin, cheekbones, and upper lip. I will first examine the nose externally and make note of deformities, deficiencies and asymmetries. Details about the shape of your nose and its relationship to the chin and lips are important and will be taken into account.

Since the nose may not be fully developed before the age of 16 or 17, I usually recommend that young adults wait until they are at least that age—and possibly older for boys—before undergoing rhinoplasty. Assuming you are in good health, there is no upper age limit for having your nose reshaped. With age, gravity and the gradual weakening of the supportive structures of the nose, the shape and position of the nose will ultimately change. Your nose may appear longer as the tip gradually droops. Thus, it is not unusual to have nasal refinements performed later in life. A simple elevation of the nasal tip will result in a younger and more attractive appearance to the nose. I am also seeing more men who want to have their noses reshaped.

> *Rhinoplasty is no longer reserved for teens today. Many women have their nose operated on or reoperated on at the time of a facelift.*

The concept of nasal refinement has changed dramatically over the past few decades. In former years, the operation was considered a "reduction rhinoplasty," thereby effectively reducing the size and projection of the nose. A large amount of cartilage was removed which led to the typical "nose job" look of the past.

Dr. Greenberg's Most Requested Near Perfect Noses

- Nicole Kidman
- Heidi Klum
- Sharon Stone
- Ashley Judd
- Sandra Bullock
- Jude Law
- Brad Pitt
- Pierce Brosnan

I limit the amount of tissue that is removed and focus more on repositioning the existing cartilage into a more pleasing shape to give a more natural looking nasal correction. Many people prefer to preserve some of the character and ethnic qualities of their natural noses while undergoing only subtle refinements. The major limitations in terms of what you can expect as a result of a rhinoplasty procedure have to do with your skin type, skin thickness, the thickness and position of your nasal bones, as well as the skill of the surgeon you select.

How We Do It

Rhinoplasty can be performed under general or local anesthesia with intravenous sedation. The incisions are usually made inside the rim of your nostrils. In some cases, tiny, inconspicuous incisions are also made across the bridge of skin separating your nostrils. The soft tissues of your nose are then separated from the underlying structures, and the cartilage and bone causing the deformity are reshaped.

The exact nature of the sculpting that is required depends on your particular problem and what you would like changed. If I am removing a hump, I may use a chisel or a rasp, then bring the nasal bones together to form a narrower bridge. Cartilage is trimmed to reshape the tip of the nose. If your nose is being reduced in size, your nasal bones will be carefully fractured inward at the conclusion of the procedure.

If your nose needs to be built up in certain areas, grafts using nasal cartilage, ear cartilage, rib cartilage or bone may be used. Other materials can also be used in the nose including synthetics like silastic implants, human tissue grafts or cartilage grafts from a tissue bank. The skin and soft tissues will redrape themselves over your new bony and cartilaginous framework. Breathing problems may be corrected by a procedure called septoplasty, in which the obstructed airway is opened.

Generally, a splint is placed on the bridge of your nose to maintain and protect the newly positioned tissues and structures. You may also have a small bandage placed under the tip of your nose. Packing or soft internal splints are sometimes placed inside the nostrils for additional support and to minimize bleeding. The two basic methods of performing a rhinoplasty include the closed and the open technique.

Closed Technique

I do most nasal surgery from inside the nose. Several incisions are made in the nostrils depending on what needs to be done. The closed technique does not require any external incisions. All incisions are made along the internal aspects of your nostril or septum. We use instruments that are passed into your nostrils to do the work of resculpting the bones, cartilage and nasal structures. This is the preferred surgical approach for people who don't require extensive reshaping, especially involving the nasal tip. The width of the base of your nose can also be reduced by removing a small amount of tissue along the inner aspect of each nostril flaring during either the open or closed technique.

Open Technique

The open technique includes an incision across the columella which is the small strip of skin that rests between your nostrils. This external scar is most visible from below. This method is most effective for complex nasal tip and septal deformities. One major advantage of this technique is the ability to completely expose the internal structures of your nose, and to place sutures precisely where they may be required. In very complex nasal deformations, we are better able to visualize the inner structures of the nose and can usually produce a better, more predictable result using many different surgical techniques. With this technique of rhinoplasty, however, the swelling in the nasal tip may take longer to subside. The external scar associated with the open technique is usually small and relatively well hidden along the underside of the nose. However, recovery and swelling may take longer with this procedure, and the tip of the nose remains swollen for longer.

The Recovery Period

If your nose is being reduced in size or is being straightened, an external splint will be applied for five days. Your nose may be packed lightly with gauze that will require removal in one to two days. (I usually do not do open rhinoplasty unless a severe deformity exists.) In most cases, the bridge of your nose and the tip will be taped to help minimize swelling. Swelling and bruising around your eyes will reach its peak after two or three days. Applying cold compresses will reduce this swelling and make you feel a bit better. If your nasal bones were fractured, you may have bloodshot eyes. Bruising usually subsides within seven days.

We recommend keeping your head elevated above the level of your heart for the first few days to reduce swelling and make breathing easier. You will be instructed not to get your splint or tape wet. You will also need to be careful about blowing your nose in the first few days to avoid bleeding. Some drainage is common during the first few days, and you will have stuffiness for several weeks.

Usually by the end of the first week splints are removed. Internal stitches are self-absorbing so they will not require removal. You will feel some pressure for several weeks, but you can usually resume light activity after a day. Activities that may cause blood to rush to your head such as bending, lifting, sex, or strenuous exercise should be avoided for several weeks after surgery as this may stimulate bleeding. Contact sports or any activity that may risk inadvertent trauma to the nose should be avoided for four to six weeks. It is important to use broad spectrum sun protection as the skin of the nose may be more prone to burning immediately after surgery.

Your nose may be numb, and the swelling will take longest (6-12 months or longer) to settle down in the tip. If your nose has been operated on previously, the swelling may take even longer to settle down completely. The thicker your skin, the longer it will take to see the final shape, especially at the tip.

Potential Pitfalls

A small amount of nasal bleeding or oozing is common after rhinoplasty. If it becomes excessive, you may be required to return to the office to have your nose repacked or the vessels cauterized. Infection is also possible but unlikely. Some irregularities of cartilage and bone are to be expected and are present in all noses. If a touch up is needed to correct small irregularities or asymmetries, it should not be done for at least six to 12 months after the initial surgery, so that all the tissues have healed.

STRAIGHT FROM THE HEART

Tiffany is 18 years old and about to begin her freshman year at college 500 miles away from home. She came to see me looking for a new nose and a fresh start.

"I hated my nose for as long as I can remember. Even when I was nine years old, I used to steal the pictures my parents took and hide them or tear them up. It was always wide, but a tennis accident early in my childhood really made the problem a lot worse. My parents never made me feel badly about myself—they actually used to tell me that my nose gave me character. For years I begged my parents to take me to see a plastic surgeon, so they would realize I was not just obsessing.

"It took a lot of crying, begging and pleading before they agreed to let me go for a consultation on my 16th birthday. So many kids I went to school with had it done. I think they finally caved when they saw my yearbook picture. I was almost frowning, and I looked like I was about to break down in tears.

"When I met Dr. Greenberg, he made me feel comfortable right away, and took the time to go over the kinds of changes he had in mind. He said he worked on a lot of girls my age, and they all dealt with a lot of torment from their classmates. I think my parents needed to hear that it was not just a shallow decision. I didn't need more convincing.

"I just started my first year at a new college and it is the most incredible feeling to have this chance to start over. No one here knows I had a nose job, and I can leave that part of my life behind me. Any shyness I used to have has disappeared. I feel confident meeting new people because I do not feel like I am being judged. Every morning I wake up and run to the mirror to make sure my beautiful new nose is still there. I almost cannot believe how great I look! My new boyfriend even tells me that my nose is one of the prettiest things about my face."

CHECKLIST

☐ Teenagers are particularly vulnerable to the agony that can accompany a bad nose.

☐ When performing rhinoplasty, I take the structure of your whole face into consideration. There is no "perfect nose" for every person.

DR. GREENBERG'S AFTER CARE

Do not take aspirin or any medications containing aspirin for three weeks after the surgery.

Swelling and bruising around the eyes is likely and may be worse the second morning after surgery. Use frozen peas or cold compress for two to three days.

Sleep on your back with your head elevated on two pillows for two days.

Eat only soft foods for twenty-four hours after your surgery.

No smoking or vitamins for at least two weeks following surgery.

Leave the dressing intact.

Your splint will be removed between five to seven days after surgery.

Most patients only require gauze under the nose for 24 hours.

You can clean dried blood from nostrils 48 hours after surgery with a Q-tip and water.

Do not lift any heavy objects.

Patient must have an escort home and someone to stay with you the night of the surgery.

No driving while taking pain medication.

You can shower 48 hours after surgery and get everything wet.

CHAPTER 9

All About Faces

Facelifts and Facial Implants

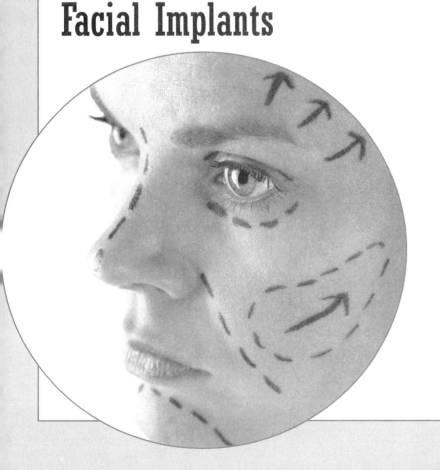

What's Hot
- The "Un-Facelift" look—where no one can tell except your hair stylist
- A little nip, a little tuck, and little scars

What's Not
- The classic wind tunnel look
- A too tight face, with old hands and flabby knees

W hen you hear the word "facelift," do you think of skin pulled so tight you can barely recognize yourself in the mirror? Many people have a very Hollywood notion of a facelift, but thanks to advances in technology, the facelift of today has become standard operating procedure. Gone are the days when face-lifts were reserved for the aging socialite or the wealthy divorcee. Now, men and women alike are turning to this surgery to restore the smooth appearance their skin once had. You may be surprised to know that a facelift is one of the easiest procedures to recover from. When done properly, it can turn back the clock by at least ten years or more.

The average age of women I see today seeking a facelift is the mid 40's. Men tend to be slightly older; around 50 is the average age. Women of color often have the good fortune of having thicker skin, so they are less likely to have premature wrinkling. They may not need a facelift until a decade later. Still, the average facelift patient is getting younger and younger, perhaps because they do not want to wait until they really need it to go in for a little rejuvenation. No one wants to look like they had a facelift.

GREENBERG'S LIST
Top Questions for Your Facelift

How long have you been doing facelift procedures? At least six years is preferable; facelifting takes years to master.

How many facelift procedures do you perform each week? At least two is preferable.

What kind of results can I expect? A well done facelift should be long lasting, at least five years or longer

What techniques do you use and why? Generally, I favor a traditional SMAS facelift approach through modified incisions. With this technique, I can limit the extent of the scars and provide a good outcome that looks natural. However, I customize my facelift operation for each individual patient.

How long will the procedure take? Two to four hours

Will I be bruised following the procedure and when will I see results? All facelift procedures will result in some bruising, which may last from one to two weeks. Most people look good at 10 days, better at three weeks, and great at six weeks.

How long does it take most of your patients to recover or return to work following facelift? Most of my patients take two weeks out of work and can return with camouflage makeup to conceal their scars.

What is the likelihood of "touch up" or "refinement" procedures? There is always a chance that a second minor procedure may be needed, but it is not common in my practice.

> *The goal is to look younger and more refreshed, without dramatic changes that give away that you had cosmetic surgery.*

Facelift surgery has become more accepted as a right of passage, rather than a frivolous self-indulgence. The ideal time for a facelift is when you think you need it, or feel ready, which varies in each individual case. Facelifts can be done successfully on people in their 70's or 80's as well, however, at that stage there is usually more to be done and results will not be as good or last as long.

HOW DO I KNOW IF I'M READY FOR A FACELIFT?

A common misconception of cosmetic surgery is that once you have a facelift, you'll have to keep having them. In fact, the opposite is true. If you ask how long a facelift will last, the answer is forever. You will always look better after having had a lift whenever you do it. Since the face continually changes with age, the benefits of having undergone surgery will ensure that you will look younger than your chronological age. Cosmetic surgery of the face involves far more than just the basic garden variety facelift today.

Aging is not limited to the surface of the skin. Time and sun damage take a toll on each layer of the skin and supportive tissues. A facelift addresses all the layers in the face.

FOUR STAGES OF AGING

1. Thickening of epidermal layer combined with diminished oil production creates a dull, lifeless and discolored appearance with little fine wrinkle lines.

2. Thinning of the dermal layer with crumbling collagen and elastic fibers leads to further wrinkle formation, sagging, crepiness, increased bruising and overall skin fragility.

3. Fat atrophy of the face leads to a sunken, tired appearance. As skin becomes less elastic, it also becomes drier. With loss of underlying support by fat padding and connective tissues, the skin begins to sag and look less supple.

4. Thickening of the muscles of expression create deeply grooved lines, folds and creases.

The Aging Face

As in the rest of the body, the appearance of the face and neck changes with age. Muscle tone is lost, causing a flabby or droopy appearance. The jowls may begin to sag, contributing to a double chin. The nose lengthens slightly and may look more prominent. There is an increase in the number, size, and color of pigmented spots on the face.

The eyebrows and eyelashes lose pigment and turn gray. The skin around the eyelids becomes loose and wrinkled, often making a crow's feet pattern. The eye socket loses some of its fat pads, making the eyes look sunken. Drooping upper eyelids can occasionally contribute to limitations in vision. The cornea may develop a grayish-white ring.

The fat pad that lies below the eye starts to thin over time, creating a sunken look to the area, and the lower eyelid tends to droop creating a "tear trough." The light that hits this area gives the illusion of a dark circle. Even the iris loses pigment, making most very elderly people appear to have gray or light blue eyes.

The bones begin to deteriorate slightly, most significantly in the inner ear which can cause changes in balance and hearing. The ears lengthen slightly caused by cartilage growth. The ear canal becomes increasingly itchy and dry. Men may find that the ear hairs become longer, coarser, and more noticeable.

Loss of teeth can make the lips look thinner. The jawbone loses bone material, decreasing the size of the lower face, and often causing the forehead, nose and mouth to look more pronounced. Gums also recede, contributing to changes in appearance of the mouth. The glands can look more pronounced on the front of the neck. Noses tend to enlarge and droop, as nasal cartilage continues to grow throughout life.

Aging doesn't happen overnight and every person's face ages differently. Some people get greater jowling earlier than others, while some have increased laxity of the neck or wrinkling on the cheeks. You don't just wake up one morning and wonder how all these changes occurred. Although they have been there all the time, you may not have noticed age-related changes until you see a recent photo.

A well-done facelift will not change your looks or make you look like a different person. Tissues are elevated to where they started out; the underlying musculature is tightened, leaving you with a refreshed appearance and sharper jawline. A facelift should do more than just tighten sagging skin. It should redrape the skin over the facial fat and muscles that have been restored to the position they held in your younger years.

When you spot someone who has undergone a facelift and looks radically different, it is usually a sign that more than just a facelift has been done. For example, adding a chin implant will make you appear slightly different than if merely a facelift is done as a stand alone procedure.

SHORTER SCARS

I am using smaller incisions now for facelifting to avoid the telltale signs of an operated on face. The skin and muscle layer (SMAS) are tightened, but shorter incisions can be used to minimize visible scars. People want to get back to their busy lives and hectic schedules quickly, and less invasive techniques are definitely what they want.

SMAS LIFT

Excess skin is removed and repositioned; the skin and the SMAS (or underlying muscle layer) are trimmed, fat is removed from under the neck, and muscles are tightened.

EXTENDED SMAS LIFT

Undermines the muscle layer to reduce sagging skin in people who have deep nasolabial (nose to mouth) folds.

SHORT SCAR FACELIFT

The modified or short scar facelift is used on younger patients with less sagging skin. The incision stops short of the hairline and extends around and in front of the sideburn area. It is also ideal for men with receding hairlines, where it is difficult to hide facelift scars.

ContourLift™

Another minimally invasive procedure involves using fine barbed sutures that attach to the underlying tissues, lifting and fixing in place the contour of the brow, midface and neck areas. By gently shifting sagging tissues in an upward direction, this technique allows the surgeon to produce a relaxed, fresh appearance. This procedure is very safe, conservative and effective, and offers natural-looking results. It works best for younger people who want a more youthful appearance, but do not want a conventional full facelift or necklift procedure. The procedure is quick and usually performed under local anesthesia, and if desired, light intravenous sedation. This should be considered a short term solution and will last two to four years, however, new devices are coming to the market that will continue to improve the threadlift procedure.

CHANGING THE SHAPE OF FACIAL BONES

Facial implant surgery is performed to build up various facial features to give your face a more balanced appearance. Facial lines and contours depend upon the skin and tissues beneath it, including the thickness and quality of fat, muscle, and bone. Implants are placed under the skin to build up contours. The regions of contour change may include the cheekbones, the jawbone and chin, as well as the lips and the nasolabial creases.

There are a wide variety of implant materials, shapes and sizes on the market including silicone based materials and human tissues. To augment a facial contour, an implant is placed deep below the skin surface and secured with permanent stitches into surrounding tissues so it doesn't move. Facial implants are typically made of solid and semi-solid materials, as opposed to gel or saline filled implants used in breast augmentation.

Another way to approach the chin and jaw is with fat transfer and other filling substances to augment the cheeks and chin, such as Restylane® and Sculptra®.

How We Do It

Chin, cheek, and jaw reshaping are outpatient procedures performed under local anesthesia with intravenous sedation or general anesthesia.

Cheek Augmentation

Malarplasty is the term for the augmentation or reshaping of the cheeks. In cheek augmentation surgery, implants are used to enhance the underlying structure, which affects the overall balance of facial features. Cheek implants may sometimes be used together with other facial implants, particularly chin implants. In some cases, prominent fat pads, called "buccal fat pads," in the cheek area may be removed to improve facial contours.

Cheek augmentation involves placing the implant over your cheekbone through an incision made inside your mouth, the outer part of your cheek, or through an opening in your lower eyelid just beneath the lower eyelash line. We create a pocket in the tissue and then place the implant directly on the cheekbone. The incisions are closed with sutures that dissolve in a week or two. At the conclusion of the surgery, your face is usually dressed with an elastic bandage to reduce swelling.

Dr. Greenberg's Most Requested Charming Cheekbones

- Michelle Pfeiffer
- Kate Hudson
- Kate Winslet
- Idina Menzel

Chin and Jaw Alterations

Adding a chin implant can be particularly effective when combined with other techniques such as face and necklifts, rhinoplasty and liposuction of the neck and jowls. Chin augmentation is usually performed by inserting a silicone implant under the skin. Most often, the incision is made beneath your chin in a natural crease and closed with sutures that are removed in five days. The access incision can also be made inside your mouth, where the lower lip meets the teeth, and then closed with resorbable sutures, but this is less commonly done today. This approach does not leave an external scar, but there may be a higher incidence of infection as the implant is placed through a contaminated field. At the end of the surgery, your chin may be taped to minimize swelling, and a compression strap is worn.

To insert jaw implants, I make incisions inside your mouth on either side of the lower lip. The implants are placed into position and the incisions are closed with dissolving sutures.

The size of the chin can also be increased by modifying the underlying bone contour. This involves using power instruments that cut the bone, and then moving the bone of the chin forward to reshape it. This operation can also be performed in conjunction with nose surgery as well as liposuction of the face and neck. Chin reduction is accomplished by cutting and repositioning the bone underneath.

Potential Pitfalls

Possible adverse consequences of facial implants include: implant extrusion, capsular contracture, asymmetry, infection, bone erosion and sensory changes. An implant that is too large or has inadequate soft tissue coverage may gradually resurface through the original access incision or through a new site. Capsular contracture, which is abnormal tightening of the scar tissue that normally forms around the implant, can cause distortion of the implant.

A facial implant is sometimes placed improperly or may shift slightly out of alignment, and a second operation may be necessary to replace it in the proper position. If an infection occurs, you are given antibiotics and the implant is temporarily removed and replaced at a later date. There may be instances where underlying bone may gradually erode and become thinner under cheek or chin implants. An area that is operated on may develop numbness that usually resolves after several months, although long-term numbness is a potential complication. In rare cases, nerve damage may occur if the implant is resting on one of the facial nerves.

What to Expect Afterward

After facial implant surgery, swelling can be significant and usually peaks 24 to 48 hours afterward. You will be instructed to keep your head elevated as much as possible in the first few days after surgery. Swelling and bruising can be minimized by an application of tape or elastic band for about a week after surgery. Applying cold compresses will also reduce swelling and discomfort.

The area may feel tight and stiff and movement of the mouth may be difficult initially following the surgery. If you have surgical incisions inside your mouth you will need to be on a liquid diet for several days. Removable sutures are used for incisions under the chin and are taken out after five to seven days.

You can return to work in one to two weeks, and resume exercise in three weeks. We recommend avoiding contact sports or any activity that may result in your face being jarred or bumped for several weeks.

STRAIGHT FROM THE HEART

Helen is a busy judge who is about to turn 50 and wants to have her face done.

"Growing up in New York City, I was very aware of image from an early age. My older sisters were real beauties, and they took great care of their skin. They taught me all their beauty secrets. About 5 years ago, my oldest sister Susan surprised my sister and I by announcing that she was going to have a facelift. We were shocked and concerned—mostly because she did not need it, and because she hated surgery of any kind. I asked her why she decided to do this and she said 'It is just time. My face needs a pick me up.'

"The truth is, I cannot see much of a difference because I think Susan looked so amazing before surgery, but she is thrilled with the way she looks. She feels the difference in her skin when she applies makeup—there is less creasing and sagging so it goes on more smoothly. Friends and relatives who have not seen her for a while come up to her and say how well she looks, but they cannot quite put their finger on what is different. Susan just smiles and winks at them and says that a few weeks in Florida did the trick.

"I recently decided to follow in the footsteps of my older sister, and go see a doctor for a consultation. I went to see Dr. Greenberg at Susan's recommendation. I had the good fortune of learning from her experience, so I knew that I wanted a natural result that did

not give away the fact that I had some work done. We also look very similar, which was an added benefit since Dr. Greenberg was already familiar with Susan's facial structure. He told me that Susan and I were both very lucky to have such good skin, and it was wise to do a little bit of improvement before it began to sag and lose its natural firmness. He explained that many women do not take care of their skin until later in life, so the damage is already done. My sisters and I always stayed out of the sun, drank plenty of water, never smoked and used a great line of skincare products. We were one step ahead of the game. Dr. Greenberg assured me that my result would be that much better for all these reasons.

"My facelift was a gift to myself. While the changes are not drastic, I noticed the improvements almost immediately. I love that Susan and I share this secret. We had a great support system in one another, and a super doctor who really knew his stuff. I sometimes joke that she was the practice and I was his masterpiece."

CHECKLIST

☐ A facelift should look natural. If someone says "Nice facelift," it probably is not.

☐ A facelift will not make you look like a different person, but it will make you look like a younger version of yourself.

☐ Do not wait until you need a facelift. The results will be so much nicer if you go in for a nip and tuck before your skin is sagging.

☐ A full facelift is not always necessary. You can get a great result with fat transfer, facial implants, fillers and Botox® if you're not ready for surgery.

☐ Every face is different, and so is every facelift.

DR. GREENBERG'S AFTER CARE

Sleep on your back with head elevated on one or two pillows for ten days following surgery.

Avoid keeping your head down for long periods of time, as the force of gravity will increase the swelling. When bending, bend at the knees.

CONTINUED

You may shower and shampoo your hair one week after surgery, keeping your head back. Do not rub over the sutured areas.

Avoid alcohol beverages for at least one week following surgery.

No strenuous activities or exercise for three weeks after surgery.

Your face may be washed in an upward position.

Normal food intake is permitted; soft foods require less chewing.

Camouflage makeup may be applied two weeks after your surgery.

Flying is not recommended until all sutures are removed in 10 days.

Avoid sun exposure for one month after surgery, and use sunscreen on any scars that are exposed.

CHAPTER 10

Smoothing Out Wrinkles and Adding Volume

Quick Fixes

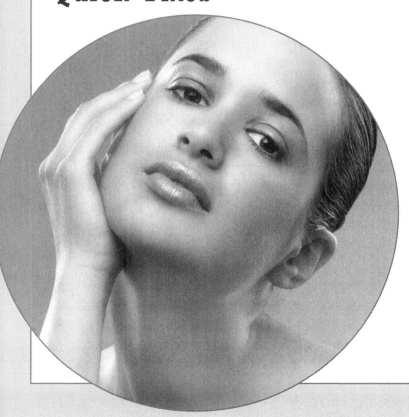

What's Hot
- Facial fullness that looks natural, soft and youthful
- Botox® to subtly raise the brows and open the eyes
- Temporary, biodegradable fillers that are safe

What's Not
- Overdone, bee-sting lips
- The frozen look of one injection too many
- Continually going back to your plastic surgeon for "just a little bit more"

Y ou do not absolutely have to go under the knife to look younger anymore. In fact, the biggest growth is in non-surgical procedures that include botulinum toxin, fillers, lasers, and peels.

The beauty of cosmetic surgery is that so many procedures are less invasive and require little or no downtime, so they fit into your lifestyle easily. There are also a number of smaller procedures that are easily performed at the same time as facial and body rejuvenation surgery to complement your overall result. These procedures can also be performed independently of a surgical procedure, particularly if you are not "ready" for surgery yet.

It is also a good idea to take your time to figure out what is best for you. You may realize surgery is the best option for you once you have gotten the maximum benefit from a wide range of fillers and injectables.

GREENBERG'S LIST
Top Filler Questions

How do I know which filler is right for me? The safest fillers are temporary and made from natural substances (fat, collagen, hyaluronic acid) that are biocompatible.

Do different fillers work best in different areas? Yes, thicker fillers are for deeper creases; thinner fillers work best for superficial lines.

How do I know how much I need of a particular filler? Let your doctor be the judge. Start small, and go back for more if you need more.

What kind of results can I expect? With most fillers, with some exceptions, results are instant.

How long will the procedure take? 15 to 30 minutes, depending on the extent of treatment and how many areas you are doing in one session.

Will I be bruised following the procedure? To avoid bruising, discontinue aspirin and anti-inflammatories, vitamin E, for one to two weeks before an injection.

How long does it take most of your patients to return to work following injections? There is very little downtime with filler treatments and Botox® and most people return to work right away or the next day. Fat injections will take longer and cause more trauma and bruising.

What is the likelihood of "touch up" or "refinement" procedures? I like to see my patients two weeks after an injection to check the results. Some times a small adjustment is needed.

MOST COMMON INJECTABLES AT A GLANCE

	HYALURONIC ACID	BOTULINUM TOXIN	HUMAN-BASED COLLAGEN	CALCIUM HYDROXY-LAPATITE	POLY–L-LACTIC ACID
PRODUCT NAME	Restylane®/ Perlane®, Juvéderm™	Botox® Cosmetic, Reloxin	CosmoDerm®, CosmoPlast	Radiesse™	Sculptra®
WHAT IT IS	A substance found in all living organisms	Botulinum toxin type A –produced by Clostridia Botulinum bacteria.	Derived from human collagen	Synthetic form of material found in bone and teeth	Ground suture material that is reconstituted with saline
HOW IT WORKS	Adds volume	Temporarily relaxes the muscle	Adds volume	Adds volume	Adds volume
INJECTION AREAS	Nasolabial folds, frown lines, crow's feet, and lips	Forehead, frown lines, crow's feet, and vertical neck bands	Nasolabial folds, frown lines, crow's feet, and lips	Nasolabial folds, frown lines,crow's feet, and lips	Nasolabial folds, corners of the mouth, cheeks

CONTINUED

RESULTS	4 months to 1 year: depending on formulation	4 months	3-4 months	1 year and possibly longer	2 years after 3 treatments
FDA STATUS	Restylane®/ Juvéderm™ are FDA approved for filling wrinkles around the nose and mouth; Perlane® is pending approval	Botox® Cosmetic is FDA approved for frown lines; Reloxin® is under investigation	FDA approved	Cosmetic use –"off-label"	Cosmetic use–"off-label"
DOWNTIME	No downtime	No downtime	No downtime	No downtime	No downtime
POSSIBLE REACTIONS	Swelling, redness, lumpiness and tenderness	Bruising, redness, droopy eyelid, flu-like symptoms, headache	Swelling, redness and bruising	Swelling, redness, bruising, and lumpiness	Swelling, redness, Bruising, lumpiness

BOTOX® AND BEYOND

Botox® has had a significant impact on the entire field of cosmetic surgery. It's safe, simple, fast and affordable—which is what everyone wants.

No other procedure has gained as much popularity as quickly as Botox® (Botulinum toxin A) Cosmetic (Allergan). Botox® is a natural purified protein that "sticks on" to nerve endings and prevents the release of the chemical transmitters that activate muscles. When injected in very low doses into specific areas of the face and neck, it inhibits the small muscles that cause frown lines, crow's feet and other wrinkles that result from making facial expressions.

If you smile, frown, or display any signs of emotion, you will likely experience facial wrinkles at some point in your life. Botulinum Toxin treatment weakens muscle activity to prevent the appearance of "dynamic" wrinkles that are caused by repeated facial expressions. Tiny amounts are injected into a specific facial muscle so only the targeted impulse stops the muscle contractions that are the underlying cause of the unwanted lines. The lines gradually smooth out because of the prolonged relaxation and the muscle blockade prevents new wrinkles from forming.

Muscles needed for important functions like eating, kissing, smiling, and eye opening are not treated, and their continued function helps to maintain a natural look. Only muscles that are treated with Botulinum Toxin are affected. I will use Botox® for treating the creases between your eyebrows and across your forehead, but other areas of your face and neck can be treated as well.

You will see improvement in a few days, but you may not see the final result for up to one week. I like to have my patients return after two weeks to make sure the look is what they expected, and do any touch-ups if needed. The effects last about four months, and repeat treatments are needed to keep the lines at bay. It is best to come back before all the muscle activity has returned to normal, so no one knows you are getting Botox®, and your lines are minimized.

Everyone responds differently to Botox®, and different areas may have longer lasting results than other areas. In order to maximize your personal results, a thorough assessment of facial wrinkles and creases is performed by examining your face at rest. I will ask you to perform a number of muscle movements including raising your eyebrows, furrowing your eyebrows, squinting your eyes, and wrinkling your nose. Based on this evaluation, I decide which areas to treat and how much Botox® to use in each area.

BOTULINUM TOXIN TYPE A

Botulinum Toxin Type A is a purified neurotoxin complex that has been used since 1980 to treat ophthalmologic muscle disorders, such as lazy eye, eye ticks, and uncontrolled blinking. A salt water solution is added before use. BOTOX® COSMETIC received approval for cosmetic use from the FDA in the spring of 2002 for glabellar creases. Treating other areas of the face and neck with Botox is considered off-label usage of the product, which means that it is not FDA approved for that site of injection. Botox® has also been FDA approved for injection into the axilla for treatment of excessive sweating.

Reloxin® (Medicis) and Puretox® (Mentor) are undergoing clinical trials in the US for a possible 2008 FDA approval.

WHERE DOES BOTOX® WORK?

Vertical lines between the brows—your "11"

Lines at the bridge of the nose

Crow's feet or squint lines

Horizontal lines on the forehead

Muscle bands on the neck

Uneven eyebrows

Popply or cobblestone chin

Chin creases

Drooping corners of the mouth

Upper lip lines

How We Do It

I perform Botox® injections in my office and it takes between 15 and 30 minutes to perform. The skin may be treated 30 to 45 minutes ahead of time with a topical anesthetic cream. A thin, fine-gauge needle like that used in acupuncture is then used to inject the Botox® through the skin and into the muscle of a specific part of the face. Crow's feet are treated with three or more injections on the side of the face close to the outer eye area or orbital rim. Horizontal forehead creases are typically treated with 10 to 16 small injections, thereby weakening rather than paralyzing the forehead muscles. The muscles that create the vertical frown lines between your eyebrows are treated with four to six small injections.

Botulinum Toxin can be used to improve but not completely get rid of the folds between the outer part of the nostrils and the corners of the lips, and the fine lines above the lips. Vertical muscle bands in the neck can also be softened. When a small amount of Botox® is injected into specific places around the eyebrows, a "chemical browlift" can be achieved which can cause a change in the eyebrow shape (rounded or peaked), and can even create a mild lifting of the eyebrows.

For deeper wrinkles, a combination of Botox® and a filler such as Restylane® can be used to achieve maximum improvement.

What to Expect Afterward

Although there is some very minor discomfort associated with the injections, there is virtually no pain afterwards. You can return to work and resume regular activities immediately after the treatment and wear makeup right away. Botox® is truly a "lunchtime" treatment.

Potential Pitfalls

Treatment with Botulinum Toxin can sometimes cause a brief head-ache and occasionally slight redness or a small bruise may occur at the injection site. A potential adverse effect is a droopy eyelid but this occurs in less than one half of one percent of people. Typically, the droop appears about five days after injection. A drooping eyelid, or ptosis, is temporary but can take up to six weeks to disappear. In some cases, you may be given prescription eye drops to speed-up resolution of the problem. Botulinum Toxin is used in higher doses in deeper muscles of the neck, and it is rare but possible to have difficulty swal-lowing temporarily after having a treatment in the neck.

If you have a neuromuscular disorder such as myasthenia gravis or are on amino glycoside antibiotics, you may be advised not to have Botulinum Toxin injections. Women who are pregnant, nursing, or who are trying to become pregnant may be advised not to be treated.

DERMAL FILLERS

Dermal fillers are injected or implanted under the skin to plump up hollow contours, soften wrinkles, and fill in furrows and some depressed scars on the face. The most popular filling substances are hyaluronic acid, collagen and fat. Thinner substances work better for fine lines and superficial wrinkles and for thin-skinned areas around your eyelids and lip lines.

Generally, thicker substances are best for deeper creases, and contouring slightly larger areas such as cheek hollows. The duration of dermal fillers depends on the formulation of the material, how deeply it is injected, and how much is used. The fillers I use are temporary so that repeat treatments will be needed.

Topical anesthetic agents are often used for numbing the area and a dental block may be utilized for very sensitive areas, like the lips, or for patients who are afraid of needles.

It is not uncommon to return to the office for touch-up injections after your initial treatment. Even if a small dose adjustment is not needed, I like to see my patients again to check the effect of the treatment.

What types of fillers are most popular?

Temporary These are the most common variety of fillers and are made from natural or synthetic materials that are broken down and resorbed by the body over time. The effects are temporary and will need to be repeated.

Permanent These fillers have synthetic components that do not get broken down by the body. They are considered permanent because the particles cannot be removed, or 'semi permanent' because the particles are suspended in a substance that gets absorbed in three to six months.

HYALURONIC ACID GEL

Hyaluronic acid is a natural polysaccharide (sugar like substance) that is commonly found in the connective tissues of the body. The source of

the material can be from animals (avian protein; i.e., roosters or poul-
try), or bacterial fermentation which is non-animal. Its normal function
in the body is to bind water and to lubricate moving parts like joints.
The most commonly used wrinkle fillers worldwide are made from
hyaluronic acid gel.

Restylane®

Restylane® (Medicis) is the most widely used hyaluronic acid gel filler
in the world. It lasts six months or longer in most cases. Because it is
a gel, it offers a soft, natural-looking correction. Restylane®, Perlane®,
and Restylane® Touch are all the same material packaged in a different particle size. Perlane® has a large particle size while the size of
Restylane® particles is small. We use the larger particles when we need
to fill deep wrinkles and the smaller ones when I need to fill superficial
ones. Restylane® is the only product presently approved by the FDA
for use in the United States; however since Perlane® and Restylane®
Touch are the exact same molecule, approval is expected shortly. We
use Restylane® to treat nasolabial creases (smile lines) and other deep
creases around the mouth and between the eyebrows when Botox® is
not effective.

Juvéderm™

Juvéderm™ (Allergan) is a homogenous gel that does not contain gel
particles. It is manufactured and is not derived from animals. Three ver-
sions are presently available and they are well suited to a broad range
of applications. There are three varieties of Juvéderm™ that were FDA
approved in 2006; Juvéderm™ 24, 24HVand 30HV. Each product varies
in the concentration of hyaluronic acid contained.

Hylaform® and Hylaform® Plus

Hylaform® and Hylaform® Plus (Allergan) are hyaluronic acids that
are derived from rooster combs. Hylaform® Plus has a larger particle
size and is designed for deeper creases. Hylaform® lasts about three or
four months.

Captique®

Captique® (Allergan) is basically the same as Hylaform® with the major difference that it is manufactured rather than harvested from rooster combs. This allows the product to be produced without any animal proteins that theoretically can cause allergic reactions. It is the same concentration and thickness as Hylaform®, and it is reasonable to assume it will have the same longevity.

Sculptra®

Sculptra® (Sanofi-Aventis) is based on a substance called poly-L-lactic acid (PLA) which occurs naturally and has been used in suture material for years. PLA stimulates production of the body's own collagen within the line or wrinkle, making the skin appear smoother and firmer. Sculptra® is reconstituted before it is injected and is most commonly used in the nasal labial folds, cheek hollows and scars. The substance is non-allergenic and typically two to three treatment sessions are recommended for best results. It is injected deeper than many other fillers, and the results are not instant. You need three treatments to get a good result.

COLLAGENS

Bovine Collagen

Zyderm® and Zyplast® (Allergan) are made from highly purified bovine dermal collagen that has been used to correct facial imperfections since the 1980's. The bovine collagen is processed to create a product that is similar to human collagen. There are three forms: Zyderm 1®, Zyderm 2®, and Zyplast®. Four weeks prior to the procedure, a test dose is administered in the forearm to determine if you have a sensitivity to the implant material. Three percent of people tested may have sensitivities. Frequently a second test dose is administered. Collagen has been largely replaced by newer substances including human collagen and hyaluronic acid gel.

Human Collagen

CosmoDerm® and CosmoPlast® (Allergan) contain human collagen that has been purified from a single fibroblast cell culture. These products contain 0.3 percent lidocaine, so additional local anesthesia is usually not required. No skin test is required because this is fashioned from human tissues rather than an animal source. CosmoDerm® and Cosmo-Plast® are injected just below the surface of the skin to fill in superficial lines and wrinkles and to define the border of the lips.

LONGER LASTING FILLING SUBSTANCES

Radiesse™

Radiesse™ (BioForm Medical) is composed of calcium hydroxyapatite, which has been used in the body for multiple applications including cheek and chin implants. Radiesse™ is a pure, synthetic calcium hydroxyl apatite composed of calcium and phosphate ions which occur naturally in the body so they are biocompatible. Radiesse™ is FDA approved only for vocal cord paralysis and urinary incontinence, however, off-label use is permitted in the US. It is ideal for use in older patients with deep folds.

ArteFill®

ArteFill® (Artes Medical) is a semi-permanent filler made up of 75 percent bovine collagen and 25 percent polymethyl-methacrylate microspheres (PMMA), which has been used in dental work, hip prostheses, and bone cement. The product is mixed with a local anesthetic, lidocaine, to numb the area to be injected. Over 3 months, the collagen fibers get absorbed, leaving the PMMA behind, which are too large to be broken down and remain permanently. It is tunneled under the skin, massaged and molded to fill the area to be treated. ArteFill® can be used for acne scars, nasolabial folds, and for filling depressions such as sunken cheeks.

Injectable Liquid Silicone

Injectable liquid silicone is a permanent filler. It is injected with a technique known as "microdroplet" to avoid lumps. It has recently had a comeback, and some plastic surgeons and dermatologists are using it as a wrinkle filler after a long hiatus. Liquid silicone is only approved by the FDA for ophthalmic uses, so cosmetic uses are considered an off-label use of an approved product. There are potential severe problems with silicone injections such as extrusion and lumpiness.

Recycling Your Own Fat

Fat is used as a filling substance in facial rejuvenation. The fat that is injected into facial areas comes from your own body, so there is no chance of an allergic reaction or "rejection." Fat can be used in higher volumes than most other injectable materials and can be used to create a fuller, more youthful appearance by reestablishing pleasing contours. Injections of fat into the deep layers of facial tissue can soften the angular, thin appearance that often accompanies aging. Fat is the first choice of material when injections of larger volumes and multiple areas are needed.

The fat must be harvested from your own body, typically from the abdomen, thighs or hips. After it is extracted, it is placed in a centrifuge to separate the fat from blood and other fluid. The fat is then packed into a syringe ready to be injected. Because fat molecules are somewhat larger than other injectable materials, it is usually injected more deeply and with a larger gauge needle.

Fat injections have a very variable life span. The fat is slowly absorbed by the body, although the amount of absorption is variable and hard to predict. Typically, more than half of the fat used in injectable treatments is absorbed with six months of the procedure, although it may last longer. Almost all people will permanently retain some of the injected fat.

I often prefer to use fat transfer techniques at the time of other facial surgery, such as eyelid, brow or facelift surgery, to enhance results, especially on a thin patient who has lost fullness in the cheeks.

LUSCIOUS LIPS

There are many options for improving the look of your lips to make them fuller and sexier. Injections or implants can enhance and improve your natural look. The upper and lower lips can be "outlined" by injecting a thin line of Restylane® or Juvéderm™ along the vermillion border and can also be made fuller with fat injections.

> **Dr. Greenberg's Most Requested Luscious Lips**
>
> - Angelina Jolie
> - Scarlett Johansson
> - Kate Beckinsale
> - Kate Bosworth

Many people say that they are afraid to have their lips enhanced because you see so many celebrities with "bee-stung" lips that look ridiculously obvious. Lip enhancement can be done in such a subtle way that no one will be able to tell that your lips have been injected at all. It can offer a very pretty and feminizing effect, especially in lips that have lost definition with age.

What to Expect Afterward

Recovery time will depend on the type and extent of the treatment and how much material is injected. Most injectable fillers have short recovery periods and you can return to work the same day or the next day. Most people experience some swelling and redness for the first 24 to 48 hours. Bruising can be minimized by avoiding the use of aspirin or aspirin-containing products for seven to ten days prior to the planned injections.

Potential Pitfalls

There may be bruising and swelling following any dermal filler treatment. You may develop asymmetries or irregularities that can usually be corrected with massage or additional injections. Some substances such as bovine collagen require pre-treatment testing for allergic reactions.

SKIN RESURFACING

Polishing down wrinkles from the top down can be done with a variety of techniques that fall under the category of skin resurfacing. Each technique accomplishes the same goal of stripping off the top layers of skin. The deeper the resurfacing, the more dramatic the result but the longer it takes to heal. If you have superficial fine lines, you will need more superficial treatments. If your lines are deeper or more coarse, you may require more aggressive peeling techniques and laser therapies.

Chemical Peels

A chemical peel involves the application of one or more exfoliating agents to the skin, causing the destruction of portions of the epidermis (outer skin layer) and/or dermis (deeper skin layer). I will choose a particular peeling agent based on your skin type and the specific problems that need to be addressed. A peel treatment begins with cleansing the skin. The face is then rinsed with water and blown-dry with a small fan. The solution is applied to the treated areas with a sponge, cotton pad, cotton swab or light brush. We apply the peeling agent so that all areas of the skin to be treated are covered evenly. The peeling solution is left in place for a few minutes and then thoroughly neutralized or removed with water.

You will be asked to limit your sun exposure for at least one month before chemical peeling, and to refrain from shaving or waxing facial areas for several days or weeks. Darker skin poses special considerations due to increased risk of undesirable skin pigmentation changes.

What are chemical peels?

Light Peels

The most commonly performed chemical peels are superficial. These formulations consist of mild chemical solutions like glycolic acid, lactic acid, and salicylic acid, which lightly peel the skin and involve almost no recovery. Salicylic acid peels treat sun damaged, thicker skin, and can also unclog pores and improve acne.

Superficial chemical peels usually take 10 to 20 minutes and these types of peels are typically done in a series to maintain the results over time. The solution used is typically adjusted for each treatment session based on your skin's response. Your face may be slightly red, and you can expect the redness to be followed by temporary flaking, dryness and scaling until your skin adjusts to the treatments. For the best results, superficial peels should be combined with an at home skin care regimen.

Medium Peels

Trichloroacetic Acid (TCA) or other solutions are used to treat pigment problems, superficial blemishes, melasma, moderate sun damage, fine lines and blotchiness. You may feel warmth or a burning sensation which is followed by some stinging. We can control the depth to which the chemical penetrates. In some cases, I may prescribe skin preparation with bleaching agents like Hydroquinone to decrease the incidence of problems with skin discoloration after the peel.

I rarely do anything deeper than a medium peel anymore. With the advent of laser technologies, most people prefer to have shorter recovery times and come back for additional treatments, rather than have a single invasive peel that may take one to three weeks to heal.

> *One of the most popular skin treatments is microdermabrasion. People love the way it makes their skin feel and the results are cumulative.*

Microdermabrasion Mania

Microdermabrasion entails treating the face with sterile micro-particles to rub off the very top skin layer, followed by removal of the sloughed skin cells. The technique exfoliates and gently resurfaces your skin and is usually performed on the face and neck. Microdermabrasion can improve rough skin texture, mild scarring, uneven pigmentation, acne lesions, blackheads, and fine wrinkles. One of the advantages of micro-dermabrasion is that it can be safely used for all skin types.

Through a wand-like hand piece, tiny aluminum oxide or salt crystals are delivered at high velocity onto the skin surface and immediately vacuumed away with the same instrument, taking the outermost layer of dead skin cells with it. The pressure can be varied to control the amount of penetration, or pass over an area several times to remove the most damaged skin. Each treatment will take about 30 to 45 minutes. A typical regimen consists of a series of four to eight treatments done at intervals of two to four weeks. Some of my patients come in every two weeks just for a light treatment to keep their skin looking smooth and clear. It also works great on chests, hands, legs, and backs.

What to Expect Afterward

Superficial peels and microdermabrasion treatments require little or no downtime. After the procedure, your skin may be coated with a mild ointment. For medium or deep peels, you may have up to ten days of crusting and peeling. You may be given an ointment to apply for seven to ten days following the peel to keep it supple and to prevent scabbing. Most people can resume their normal activities immediately after superficial treatments, and within four to ten days following aggressive procedures, when the new skin has emerged.

With all peels and lasers, you should avoid direct sun exposure for several months to protect the newly formed layers of skin and minimize pigmentary changes.

Potential Pitfalls

The possible adverse consequences following chemical peels include infection, dermatitis, scarring, and pigmentary changes. The skin color may become lighter or darker. Darker skin types are at a higher risk for darker pigmentation but may also suffer from a lightening of the skin color. Any peel carries the risk of cold sores in people who have a history of recurring fever blisters or herpes simplex outbreaks.

STRAIGHT FROM THE HEART

Charlie is a 30-something fashion stylist in Manhattan who has never had cosmetic surgery, but wanted to add some volume to her face.

"I was not big on cosmetic surgery, but I am in a business where beauty is the be all and end all. Working with the hippest, most attractive, not to mention, young and skinny, girls in Manhattan can do a number on your self-esteem. Every day these hot young models, actresses, and ladies who lunch come to my studio and I make them look even better than they already do. I was actually shocked when one rising 'It girl' just casually mentioned during a fitting that she had Botox® twice a year to fend off the 'wrinkles' she already started seeing, and was going for lip injections as well—even though she already had the prettiest mouth I had ever seen.

"This same client and I became close friends, and over the next year or so, she taught me a lot about the 'beauty secrets' of the in-crowd. I could not believe how many young celebs were having work done, and the models I saw didn't all look so perfect without a little help here and there. It was a lot more than just injections—we are talking breast implants, tummy tucks, and liposuction on basically every inch of their size zero bodies. Compared to some of these women, her injections were less of a big deal than I thought.

"Of course, I got curious and went to see what I could do for myself. Dr. Greenberg was the second and last doctor I saw. I took a look at before and after pictures of some women my age. I asked a million and one questions. Before I put anything in my body I wanted to know where it came from and what it would do to me. I was actually the most interested in Restylane® for my nasolabial folds, and while I was at it, a little bit for my lips. I will never be Angelina Jolie, but I can still look sexy. I got myself a little holiday present I could enjoy all year round."

CHECKLIST

☐ Fillers come in many forms, and are great for a little touch up.

☐ If you cannot handle a needle, you cannot handle a scalpel. Start small and work your way up to the more involved procedures as you need them.

☐ Know the difference between permanent and semi-permanent fillers.

☐ Take into account the expense of upkeep injections over time. It is something to consider when you are deciding if surgery may eventually be right for you.

☐ From chemical peels to microdermabrasion, skin resurfacing is a simple way to get glowing.

CHAPTER 11

Laser Services

All About Hair Removal, Red Veins, Brown Spots

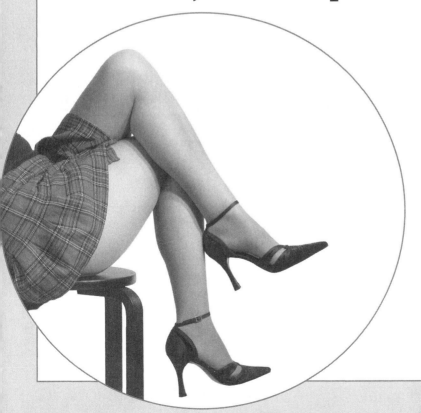

What's Hot
- Skin tightening technologies for the face, neck, and eyelid area
- Skin tightening technologies for tummies, thighs, and arms
- Laser treatments for the body

What's Not
- Peel overload
- Stretched faces that have a shine
- Hitting the tanning booth or the beach without protection after you have lasered away your old sun damage

The power of lasers is truly amazing. Years ago, the prospect of light sources being used to get rid of ugly veins, discolorations and even unsightly hair, would have sounded like science fiction. Today, state-of-the-art lasers offer patients fairly painless vein removal, and removal of sun spots, rosacea, and brown spots. It is a time and cost-effective alternative to the annoying upkeep of waxing, shaving and other methods of hair removal. You can kiss your discolorations goodbye. Say hello to smooth, spotless skin for years to come!

GREENBERG'S LIST
Top Laser Questions

How long have you been doing laser procedures? At least three years is preferable.

How many laser procedures do you perform each week? At least 10 is preferable.

What types of lasers do you use? I use several lasers and devices to address different conditions. For example, the most popular device we use is an IPL.

How do I know which laser is best for which procedure? This is where you have to trust the doctor you have chosen, and let him or her decide which laser is right for you.

What kind of results can I expect? Most of the devices we use provide a subtle improvement after each treatment, and will have to be repeated in a course of three to five or more.

How long will the procedure take? Light based therapies are done very quickly—20 to 45 minutes for a treatment. Skin tightening techniques take longer to do.

Will I be bruised following the procedure and when will I see results? In most cases, there is no bruising, but there may be slight redness or swelling in more sensitive skin types. The response is very variable.

How long does it take most of your patients to recover or return to work following laser therapy? Most of the treatments I do can be performed in the office and patients return to work right away or the next day without any disruption to their daily schedule.

LASERS & LIGHT SOURCES

A laser is a high-energy beam of light that can selectively direct its energy into the tissue. These beams can be targeted to a specific point and varied in intensity and in duration of emitted pulses. In addition to skin resurfacing, lasers can be used to treat numerous skin conditions including broken capillaries, acne scars, unwanted hair, tattoos, discolorations, and age spots. People with darker skin types have a higher risk of pigmentation changes after laser treatment.

Different types of lasers are suited to treating specific problems. Non-ablative devices are the most popular, and these penetrate through to the layers beneath to boost collagen production, which gives the skin a fresher, plumper, more youthful appearance. Most people do not want to take the time out of their lives to have deeper resurfacing procedures any more, such as phenol peels or carbon dioxide laser. They prefer to have smaller treatments more often to produce the same or similar results.

Fraxel®

The newest buzz in laser technology is called fractional resurfacing or Fraxel® (Reliant). It will probably replace deep treatments except for the most severe wrinkles. This device removes old skin cells as it penetrates the skin. The consensus is that fractional resurfacing is intermediary between ablative and non-ablative technologies. Fractional resurfacing offers a greater degree of precision than many other lasers: it treats very small areas of the skin but leaves the surrounding tissue intact. This "fractional" treatment allows the skin to heal rapidly than and it allows the body to create new, healthy tissue to replace old and damaged skin. The treatment can be done in the office with only topical anesthesia. Most patients experience a mild sunburn sensation for a few hours and the skin remains pink for five to seven days following treatment. There is typically a minimal degree of swelling that lasts for two or three days. Epidermal regeneration is rapid, often beginning within 24 hours of the treatment. Following treatment, it is important to use sunblock and allow your skin to heal. In most cases, three to four treatments are necessary, and it can be used on the face, neck, chest, as well as hands. We have seen good results for pigment, melasma and skin tone and texture and possibly acne scars, but this is not a home run for wrinkles yet. Still, it has some of the same risks of other lasers.

Titan®

Titan® (Cutera®) uses broad spectrum infrared light to heat the deep layers of the dermis and renew collagen in the skin. As a result of this deep target, surface skin is not damaged. Topical numbing cream is used to dull sensation. While you may experience slight redness after the procedure, it should disappear in an hour or so, and any swelling should disappear after about a day. The procedure takes about ten minutes to perform and will not prevent you from continuing your daily tasks, so you can return to work afterward if you wish. You will begin to see results after three to eight months as it takes time for the collagen to regenerate. It is most commonly used to target wrinkles and sagging skin on the face, forehead, cheek, jowls, neck and abdomen.

NON-ABLATIVE LASERS

This class of lasers does not produce a deep burn and they give a minimally invasive treatment that improves skin texture and tone by stimulating new collagen in the skin to smooth it out from underneath. These treatments do not destroy outer tissue as they work their way down to stimulate collagen growth in the dermis. Each device delivers controlled energy to the skin in slightly different ways, but the process is gradual and the softening of wrinkles occurs over time as the rejuvenated skin fibers reach the skin surface. Treatments are usually repeated every four to six weeks over a six month period to maximize new collagen formation.

Since non-ablative lasers often have a very long wavelength, they are relatively safe for a variety of skin types. A topical anesthetic may be all that is necessary to numb the skin for more superficial procedures. Most people will see an improvement in 30 days and may continue to see improvements for up to 90 days. The newly formed collagen will then age at the normal rate and you can repeat the procedure for maintenance as needed. These are great for mild wrinkling.

Intense Pulsed Light Sources (IPL)

These versatile light sources work by creating a wound in the small blood vessels found in the dermis that causes collagen and blood vessels under the top layer to constrict. The light energy is delivered through the skin, removing facial redness, erasing pigmented spots, reducing pore size and minimizing fine lines. A series of five or six photo facial treatments are given at three to four week intervals. There may be some minor discomfort similar to a rubber band snapping against the skin. You can return to work or resume normal activities immediately after the procedure.

After one or two treatments, your skin will have more even tone and texture. If you have rosacea and facial flushing, you can expect to see a reduction in redness after each treatment. This treatment is good for fine lines particularly around the eyes and mouth, shallow acne scars, age spots, broken blood vessels, enlarged pores, and chronic facial redness. It can also be used to treat sun damaged areas on the neck, arms and chest, and hands. This works best for patients with early mild wrinkling and sun damage (30's to 50's).

By far, this is the most popular skin treatment in my practice. My patients love the way their skin looks, and the fact that there is no downtime and no one has to know they are having it done are also pluses.

Photo Dynamic Therapy

Laser-assisted photodynamic therapy (PDT) is being used as an alternative to freezing with liquid nitrogen and topical chemotherapy for brown spots called actinic keratoses. The treatment works in two stages. First, a light-activated aminolevulinic acid is applied to the skin. About 14 hours later, a pulsed-dye laser light seeks out and selectively treats only the acid covered areas. PDT therapy may also be used for facial rejuvenation and acne.

LED Technology

This is a very hot technology because it is totally non-invasive. Photo-modulation refers to using low-energy light to accelerate or inhibit cell activity. Basically, during the treatment, you sit in front of a panel of low level light emitting diodes (LED's). Unlike laser technology that relies on high-powered coherent light to create heat energy, LED photo-modulation triggers the body to convert light energy into cell energy without damaging the tissues with heat. IPL (intense pulsed light) is a variation of this theme. Both are gentle, require multiple treatments to see very subtle results, and require little or no downtime. LED's can also be used to reduce redness and inflammation after filler treatments and deeper resurfacing.

SKIN TIGHTENING

Using radio frequency waves or infrared energy to tighten loose skin on the neck, face and body areas works by delivering deep intense heat into the skin without injury to the epidermis. There are several systems currently on the market that work in different ways. One treatment may be sufficient depending on the area, but in some cases, multiple treatments may be done for best results.

Thermage®

Thermage® radiofrequency technology is part of our combination therapy menu of non-invasive facial rejuvenation. It is primarily a tech-nique for lifting and tightening, not for wrinkle or pigment reduction. Thermage® stimulates the gradual growth of new collagen, temporar-ily reduces wrinkles, and renews facial contours. I use it to tighten the eyelid skin, raise the eyebrows, and tighten the forehead. A single Thermage® treatment tightens your existing collagen and stimulates new collagen growth. Improvements are both immediately visible and continue up to six months. Thermage® works on your entire face—forehead, eyes, nasolabial folds, jaw line, jowls and the area under your chin.

Thermage® treatments require no incisions or downtime. They can provide a more youthful facial appearance, but the results generally last around two years—not nearly as long as an actual facelift. It does, however, last longer than injectable fillers. Thermage® stimulates the gradual growth of new collagen, temporarily reduces wrinkles, and renews facial contours.

Skin tightening offers patients the advantage of a subtle lifting effect without the risks, recovery and scars of traditional surgery.

There had been so much hype and discussion about how much the Thermage® procedure hurts that many patients are very surprised that the most current techniques are not very uncomfortable and that there is no downtime.

ReFirme™

ReFirme™ (Syneron) is one of the newest non-invasive wrinkle treatment and skin tightening for the neck, face, and body. The advantage of this technology is speed: it has a pulse repetition rate of one pulse per second, which makes it faster, less painful, and more effective than other comparable devices.

HAIR REMOVAL TECHNOLOGIES

Laser hair removal has become one of the most common cosmetic procedures performed in the United States. Using state-of-the-art laser hair removal techniques to gently remove unwanted hair, we can put an end to routine shaving and waxing. Your skin will look and feel smoother after each treatment. Laser hair removal is less painful and uncomfortable than many other hair removal treatments, including electrolysis or even waxing.

Laser hair removal utilizes beams of highly concentrated light to selectively penetrate hair follicles. The energy gets absorbed by the pigment in the hair follicles and to destroy the hair. The newest technologies have made the procedure safer for patients with darker skin and those of color. The laser device we use has a wide beam to easily treat larger areas such as the back, shoulders, arms, legs, as well as the chin and lip. Most people will require a series of at least three treatments to achieve a long term or permanent reduction of unwanted hair.

VANISHING SPIDER VEINS

Unsightly veins can show up on your legs, face, and chest. They are sometimes caused by sun damage and are also a sign of aging skin. Spider vein removal by laser provides a safe and effective, non-surgical treatment option for the removal of spider veins. Vein removal treatments deliver a precise dosage of energy to each vein, with minimal risk to the skin. During your treatment, light energy is delivered through a special hand piece with filters to the targeted vein, in a series of short and/or long pulses. The light energy is absorbed by the blood vessels. This heat absorption gradually shuts down the vein. There is little discomfort for most patients and significant improvement can be seen after just one or two treatments. We use the Altus® laser, one of the most advanced, gentlest and safest lasers on the market today.

How We Do It

The laser and light source will be set with the best parameters for each individual based on their skin color and what we are treating. Depending on the laser or light source, either a cold gel or a special cooling device will be used to protect the outer layers of the skin. This also helps the laser light penetrate further into the skin. We then apply a pulse of light to the treatment area. When the procedure is finished, it is common for the area treated to have some mild redness for 12 to 24 hours. At the conclusion of the procedure, ice is applied to the area treated

What to Expect Afterward

The healing time depends on the depth to which the laser penetrated.

It may take a week or more for the skin to reepithelize. Absolutely NO sun exposure will be allowed for four to eight weeks, and broad spectrum sunscreen with UVA and UVB block should be worn at all times.

Technology changes constantly and new lasers and light sources continually come to market offering more effective and safer options. Often, a combination of devices may be used to effectively treat specific conditions, and a variety of different treatments may effectively accomplish the same goals. It is nearly impossible for a consumer to keep up to date with new technologies as they are introduced, and to be able to evaluate which is appropriate for your particular skin type and concern. The best advice is to select a qualified plastic surgeon you trust and let his or her recommendations guide you, rather than to be persuaded by individual technologies that you read about in magazines or online.

Potential Pitfalls

Any laser treatment may lead to blisters, burns, scarring, and pigmentation changes, in addition to the risk of cold sores in patients who have a history of recurring fever blisters or herpes simplex. People with darker skin color are more prone to blotchiness and permanent skin darkening. Sometimes an inconspicuous spot test behind your ear is a good idea to determine if you are a good candidate for the procedure.

> *Even laser hair removal is a medical procedure. Don't take any risks by having treatments done by untrained technicians without a doctor on site.*

STRAIGHT FROM THE HEART

Andrew is a 63-year-old builder who spent too many years in the California sun. He came to me to get rid of some prominent age spots.

"I confess: I was a sun worshipper. When I was growing up surfing, swimming, and laying in the sun no one knew how dangerous it was. I never wore sunscreen. I burned to a crisp too many times. That

is what we did in California. It was always summer. There were no signs of danger.

"As an adult I started to notice brown spots on my skin. My wife is from New England and she has a very fair complexion. There was a big difference in our skin tones, and as I watched the news and read more stories of skin cancer, I started to wonder about my own risks. I spoke to my cousin who is a doctor. As kids we were unaware of the need for taking care of our skin.

"My cousin told me about all of the new technologies and mentioned that lasers were very popular for fixing skin problems. He sent me some literature on sun spots and age spots. I told him I would only consider doing something about the spots if it was quick and did not force me to stop my life. He assured me this would be very low maintenance, and I should see a plastic surgeon.

"I visited Dr. Greenberg in Manhattan and asked him about lasers. He said it was a good choice for me. The main problem areas for me were my face, shoulders, and arms. The procedure was quick and practically painless. Dr. Greenberg said I would need to have about five treatments to get rid of most of the sun damage. The brown spots faded a little bit with each session. Even at 63, I learned a lesson. It may be too late to undo all the damage I did to my skin as a kid, but if I can catch something before it starts that is a step in the right direction.

"Now both my wife and I do skin checks every few months, just to make sure we are healthy. We want to be sure we are taking care of ourselves."

CHECKLIST

- [ ] There are different types of lasers for different types of skin problems. As always, do your homework so you are up to date on the latest technologies.
- [ ] Lasers are ideal for hair removal in areas that are a nuisance to maintain—such as the bikini line or upper lip.
- [ ] If you have dark skin, you should do a spot test to make sure lasers will not cause permanent discoloration.

CHAPTER 12

How to Get the Best Results

From Fillers to Facelifts and Beyond

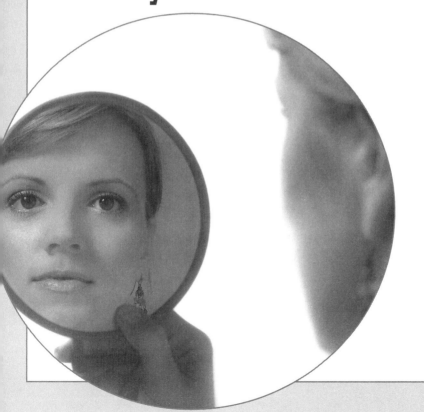

W hether you are preparing for a facelift or a Botox® injection, you should be as comfortable as possible before and after the procedure. This chapter will give you all the pointers you need to make your image enhancement a pleasant experience overall.

NEW YOU IN REVIEW: Potential Pitfalls
Source: The National Women's Health Information Center

PROCEDURE	RISKS
Breast augmentation Breasts are enlarged by placing an implant behind each breast.	• Implants can rupture, leak, and deflate • Infection • Hardening of scar tissue around implant, causing breast firmness, pain, distorted shape, or implant movement • Bleeding • Pain • Nipples may get more or less sensitive • Numbness near incision • Blood collection around implant/incision • Calcium deposits around implant • Harder to find breast lumps
Breastlift Extra skin is removed from the breast to raise and reshape breast.	• Scarring • Skin loss • Infection • Loss of feeling in nipples or breast • Nipples put in the wrong place • Breasts not symmetrical

CONTINUED

Breast reduction Fat, tissue, and skin are removed from breast.	• If nipples and areola are detached, may lose sensation and decreased ability to breastfeed • Bleeding • Infection • Scarring • Harder to find breast lumps • Poor shape, size, or position of nipples or breasts
Eyelid surgery Extra fat, skin, and muscle in the upper and/or lower eyelid is removed to correct "droopy" eyelids.	• Blurred or double vision • Infection • Bleeding under the skin • Swelling • Dry eyes • Whiteheads • Can't close eye completely • Pulling of lower lids • Blindness
Facelift Extra fat is removed, muscles are tightened, and skin is rewrapped around the face and neck to improve sagging facial skin, jowls, and loose neck skin.	• Infection • Bleeding under skin • Scarring • Irregular earlobes • Nerve damage causing numbness or inability to move your face • Hair loss • Skin damage

CONTINUED

Facial implant Implants are used to change the nose, jaws, cheeks, or chin.	• Infection • Feeling of tightness or scarring around implant • Shifting of implant
Forehead lift Extra skin and muscles that cause wrinkles are removed, eyebrows are lifted, and forehead skin is tightened.	• Infection • Scarring • Bleeding under skin • Eye dryness or irritation • Impaired eyelid function • Loss of feeling in eyelid skin • Injury to facial nerve causing loss of motion or muscle weakness
Lip augmentation Material is injected or implanted into the lips to create fuller lips and reduce wrinkles around the mouth.	• Infection • Bleeding • Lip asymmetry • Lumping • Scarring
Liposuction Excess fat from a targeted area is removed with a vacuum to shape the body.	• Baggy skin • Skin may change color and fall off • Fluid retention • Shock • Infection • Burning • Fat clots in the lungs • Pain • Damage to organs if punctured • Numbness at the surgery site • Heart problems • Kidney problems • Disability • Death

CONTINUED

Nose surgery	
Nose is reshaped by resculpting the bone and cartilage in the nose.	• Infection • Bursting blood vessels • Red spots • Bleeding under the skin • Scarring
Tummy tuck	
Extra fat and skin in the abdomen is removed, and muscles are tightened to flatten tummy.	• Blood clots • Infection • Bleeding • Scarring • Fluid accumulation

WHAT IS IT?	RISKS
Botox® injection	
Botox is injected into a facial muscle to paralyze it, so lines don't form when a person frowns or squints.	• Face pain • Muscle weakness • Flu-like symptoms • Headaches • Loss of facial expression • Droopy eyelids • Asymmetric smile • Drooling
Fat injection	
Fat from your thigh or abdomen is injected into facial wrinkles, pits, or scars.	• Contour problems • Swelling • Infection • Redness
Hyaluronic acid injection	
This gel is injected into your face to smooth lines, wrinkles, and scars	• Swelling • Infection • Redness • Tenderness • Acne • Lumps • Risks unknown if used in combination with collagen
Laser hair removal	
Laser light is passed over the skin to remove hair.	• Hair regrowth • Scarring • Change in skin color

CONTINUED

Laser skin resurfacing Laser light is used to remove wrinkles, lines, age spots, scars, moles, tattoos, and warts from the surface of the skin.	• Burns • Scarring • Change in skin color • Infection • Herpes flare-up (fever, facial pain, and flu-like symptoms)
Sclerotherapy A solution is injected into spider and varicose leg veins (small purple and red blood vessels) to remove the veins.	• Blood clots • Color changes in the skin • Vein removal may not be permanent • Scarring
Chemical Peel A solution is put onto the face (or parts of the face) that causes the skin to blister and peel off. It is replaced with new skin.	• Whiteheads • Infection • Raised scarring • Allergic reaction • Cold sores • Color changes or blotchiness • Heart problems

Whew! It's finally over and you did great. Along with your new look is a new and improved self-image and outlook. You don't need a million dollars to have your own "extreme makeover." To further boost your self-confidence, use your cosmetic surgery as a stepping stone to a lifetime of beauty and health.

THE SCIENCE OF ANTI-AGING

Anti-aging is for real. We can't stop the aging process, but we can definitely slow it down.

Plastic surgeons are not only interested in helping patients look better, but also helping them feel better. It's easy to dismiss some anti-aging research as junk science unsupported by solid clinical data, however, I am following the ongoing research in this field.

The field of anti-aging is very complex and rapidly evolving as new discoveries are made and research is conducted. In the areas of nutritional supplements, vitamins, minerals, and herbs, many conflicting opinions exist with different researchers and clinicians advocating different combinations of supplements and nutrients. There is no definitive evidence that any one particular combination of nutrients, supplements and vitamins is the answer to aging.

In general terms, achieving good health, longevity, and well-being require a comprehensive lifestyle approach. Our health is mostly determined by the lifestyle we lead. The majority of healthy choices are basic common sense that is obvious to all of us; for example: the importance of not smoking, drinking alcohol only in moderation, exercising regularly, avoiding stressful situations whenever possible, eating a healthy, balanced diet, and avoiding UV rays. Did you realize that smokers have a nearly five times greater chance of having a roadmap of wrinkles than those who don't smoke?

Anti-aging medicine is part of an overall strategy for improving patients' quality of life. There is every reason to be optimistic that continuing progress in the biomedical sciences will contribute to even longer and healthier lives in the future.

Genetics

While our genetic makeup is pre-determined, lifestyle, nutrition, and other factors controlled by us can radically affect the way our genes are expressed.

Hormones

A growing body of scientific evidence has shown that many hormones decline with age, and that these declines can result in many of the signs of aging. The first to be recognized is the decline in estrogen and progesterone production in women called 'menopause.' The other hormones that are well-documented to decline are testosterone in men (and, in women too), growth hormone, and the adrenal hormone

DHEA. The decline in these hormones starts much earlier and is more gradual. Melatonin also declines in many individuals.

The blood levels of other hormones can actually increase with aging. Tissue resistance to insulin can result in an increase in fasting levels and the levels in response to a meal. This can lead to an increased risk of diabetes, cardiovascular disease and cancer. Similarly, our bodies' response to stress can result in prolonged elevations of cortisol, which can wreak havoc on body composition, brain function and immune system function.

Several hormones, including growth hormone, testosterone, estrogen and progesterone, have been shown to improve some of the physiological changes associated with human aging. Under careful supervision some hormone supplements can be very beneficial. No hormone has been proven to slow, stop or reverse the aging process. Hormone supplements should not be used unless they are prescribed by a medical doctor.

GREAT SKIN

What's My Type?

There is no such thing as a healthy tan. A tan is your skin's reaction to damage that's been inflicted on it by the sun. You may think a golden glow hides your imperfections, but sun exposure actually triggers oil production, clogs your pores, and prematurely ages your skin. In order to keep your skin looking healthy, you need to know about your specific skin type.

This will allow you to tailor your sun protections, and cleansing and treatment regimens to achieve the most effective results and the most beautiful complexion. Generally, the lower your number on the scale below, the more protection you need from environmental abuse and the earlier you will start to see visible signs of aging.

FITZPATRICK SKIN TYPE CHART	
TYPE	**DESCRIPTION**
I	Never tans, always burns (Extremely fair skin, blonde hair, blue/green eyes)
II	Occasionally tans, usually burns (Fair skin, sandy to brown hair, green/brown eyes)
III	Often tans, sometimes burns (Light to medium skin, brown hair, brown eyes)
IV	Always tans, never burns (Medium complexion or olive skin, brown/black hair, dark brown/black eyes)
V	Rarely burns (Dark brown skin, black hair, black eyes)
VI	Never burns (Black skin, black hair, black eyes)

Obagi®

For people who want to try an effective clinical skincare solution, we have been very pleased with the results we can achieve with the Obagi® System. The products are able to transform common skin conditions at the cellular level to actually make skin look and feel healthier.

Obagi® Nu-Derm System helps to accelerate cellular turnover for skin with moderate to severe sun damage. It contains Tretinoin and Hydroquinone 4 percent to combat the tell-tale signs of aging such as dark spots and loss of elasticity.

Obagi®-C Rx System adds brightness for skin with mild to moderate sun damage. The Professional-C Serums offer highly potent vitamin C for maximum daily anti-oxidant protection.

Obagi® Blue Peel System is a peel we offer that is used in conjunction with the Obagi® Nu-Derm System, for people with severe hyper-pigmentation and acne scarring.

GREENBERG'S LIST OF THE TOP 10 SIGNS OF AGING SKIN

1. Blotchy complexion

2. Enlarged pores

3. Redness, broken capillaries

4. Dry rough patches

5. Hyperpigmentation, age spots, dark patches

6. Lines and wrinkles

7. Sagging eyes, jowls, and neck

8. Sallow appearance

9. Enlarging growths or moles

10. Loss of radiance

EATING FOR HEALTH

You try to eat right, but if you eat out regularly, or skip meals and snack on junk food, you may not be getting all the nutrients your body needs to thrive. To keep your skin looking young, key players are selenium, vitamins C and E. Vitamins A, B, C, D, E and K, folic acid, zinc, selenium and essential fatty acids all contribute to the skin's overall health. They act as anti-oxidants, scavenging for harmful byproducts in the body and boosting the immune system or promoting healthy cell growth.

Proper nutrition and exercise is important for healthy skin as well as overall good health. Exercise stimulates your metabolism, causes you to sweat, and increases lymphatic drainage, which keeps your skin healthy and clean. When nutrients are ingested and absorbed into your bloodstream, they are sure to be delivered to your skin cells. Nutrition has an effect on the mechanisms of aging of the body as a whole. Inhibiting these mechanisms slows down the aging process, including the aging of the skin. Nutrients and foods that benefit your skin also benefit other bodily functions.

Start by critically assessing your nutritional habits and try to fill the gaps first with food, and secondly with supplements. You need a good multi-vitamin to keep skin healthy.

Free radicals are the result of oxygen molecules being oxidized, but they can also be created by exposure to various environmental factors, smoking and UV radiation. Free radicals are known as one of the primary factors that accelerate the aging process. They are common in all people, and the body can, for the most part, defend itself with anti-oxidants that are found naturally in the body and that serve as free radical scavengers. These anti-oxidants can be used up very quickly which is why taking additional anti-oxidants in supplement form is useful.

SMILE REJUVENATION

A stunning smile can disarm everyone you come in contact with, and it is one of the first things people notice about you. Even a perfect smile will deteriorate as you get older. As you age, the outer layer of enamel on your teeth gets worn away. Eventually it reveals the darker tissue underneath, at the center of your tooth around the nerves and blood vessels. If you have discolored teeth, but are otherwise happy with your smile, bleaching may be all you need.

Whitening Up

Although there are many products and methods available, teeth whiteners may not correct all types of discoloration. For example, yellowish hued teeth will probably bleach well, brownish-colored teeth may bleach less well, and grayish-hued teeth may not bleach well at all. Your dentist may suggest a procedure that can be done in his or her office. During chairside bleaching, your dentist will apply either a protective gel to your gums or a rubber shield to protect the oral soft tissues. A bleaching agent is then applied to the teeth, and a special light may be used to activate it. Bleaching solutions contain peroxide(s), which actually bleach the tooth enamel. Peroxide-containing whiteners typically come in a gel and are placed in a mouthguard. Your dentist can make a custom-fitted mouthguard for you that will fit your teeth precisely. Over the counter methods don't work very effectively.

Porcelain Veneers

So many of my patients will invest in having their faces lifted and bodies resculpted, but overlook the importance of great looking teeth in the big picture. Gaps in your teeth or stains, misaligned and crooked teeth can be beautifully transformed through state-of-the-art porcelain veneers. Porcelain veneers can take ten years off your smile and can last 10 to 20 years. Veneers are thin, custom-made shells crafted of tooth-colored materials designed to cover the front side of teeth. They are customized from a model provided by your dentist. With porcelain veneers, the gold standard in the cosmetic dentist's arsenal, virtually anything can be done to improve a smile. They are like little shells that wrap around the tooth to create different shapes and varying shades for a totally flawless yet natural look. Laminates usually require two office visits. The teeth will be prepared and an impression made during the first visit, which can take one to four hours. The laminates will be fitted and inserted at the second visit, which may also take the same amount of time.

Orthodontics

With orthodontics, spaces between teeth are closed, and the results are generally permanent. The process requires six to thirty-six months for most adults. Retainers frequently have to be worn at night for many years, at least a few nights a week, possibly indefinitely, to maintain tooth alignment. An alternative to traditional orthodontia is Invisalign®, which uses a series of clear plastic, removable aligners to straighten teeth gradually, without metal or wires. The plastic trays, which are custom-made and resemble teeth-whitening trays, work by moving your teeth incrementally. These aligners move teeth through the controlled force, but the main advantage is that they are nearly invisible, removable, and very comfortable.

FINISHING TOUCHES

Your results are only as good as the upkeep. Maintenance after any cosmetic procedure is needed to maximize the effects.

How many times have you seen an incredibly successful makeover on television, and a few months later the cameras follow up and discover a less glamorous looking woman? I always tell my patients to remember that no procedure is a cure-all, and the rest is up to them.

But you can enhance your looks forever with some strategic planning. All of my patients meet with our aesthetician before and after a cosmetic procedure. It is a chance to learn the trade secrets of makeup, camouflage, and overall enhancement, to maximize your surgical and non-surgical results. I can work wonders for you in my office, but once you leave, it is up to you to stay looking great.

STRAIGHT FROM THE HEART

Trish is a comedian and aspiring actress who truly has something to smile about with her clear skin.

"I am in the business of making people laugh. That means when I am on stage at a comedy club everyone is looking straight at me. They are judging everything about me: my sense of humor, my clothes, and especially my skin. I used to make jokes about my zits which accounted for a good 25 percent of my material. I can make fun of myself with the best of them, so it always went over well with the crowds.

"Once I started branching out in to acting, it was a whole different world for me. I was competing with near perfect people with flawless complexions. So I dipped into my savings, and started asking around for referrals to a good doctor.

"My agent suggested that I go to see Dr. Greenberg. His aesthetician put me on a strict skincare regimen and he gave me a prescription for Avage®. She suggested that I have a few mild peels to even out my texture and purge my clogged pores. After a few weeks, my eruptions were under control, finally. You cannot imagine the satisfaction I felt in my next round of headshots. It was like night and day. I may be an out of work actress, but I am an out of work actress with clear skin for the first time since I hit puberty!"

CHECKLIST

☐ Get ready for your close-up—a great smile is the perfect finish for your cosmetic makeover.

☐ Learn the secrets of looking good to increase the longevity of your procedure of choice.

THE FUTURE OF COSMETIC SURGERY

New techniques will continue to be developed as demand for safer, faster and better procedures grows. Surgical procedures such as face-lifts, which are performed with scalpel, will become less invasive in the future. Recovery times will be quicker and scarring will be less visible, which will attract more people to having things done. Tissue engineering is making great strides in developing tissues in a laboratory that can be used as replacements for diseased body parts.

I am excited about what the future holds for plastic surgeons and for my patients. The possibilities are endless.

Appendix

THE BRIDE TO BE'S COUNTDOWN TO "I DO"

Brides are everyday women on display, which means they have the same concerns as everyone else, with more of an immediate reason to feel self-conscious about their appearance. Smile lines, wrinkles, and excess areas of fat are target areas in preparation for the big day. It is no secret that brides still hit the gym for weeks and months before the wedding date, but they don't stop there. It's about making a statement that she is the most beautiful woman in the room, and capturing magazine quality photos when the camera is unforgiving. The modern bride won't settle for less than perfection, especially on her big day.

As a bride, you want to make sure you give yourself enough time to heal so you can glide into the wedding hall calmly and at your absolute best.

Greenberg's Bridal Timetable	
PROCEDURE	TIMETABLE
Facials, microdermabrasion, chemical peels	Start 3 months before
Botox® for wrinkles	3 weeks before
Restylane® to fill out lips	3-4 weeks before
Breast Augmentation	4-6 weeks before
Liposuction	4-6 weeks before
Rhinoplasty	6-8 weeks before
Facelift, Eyelids, Browlift	6-8 weeks before

POST PREGNANCY TUNE UP

BREASTS Inadequate breast volume may be acquired after pregnancy, breast feeding, and significant weight loss. Pregnancy with or without breast feeding can lead to deflated breasts that were previously of adequate size. Caution should be exercised if you plan to have more children and/or breast feed.

TUMMY Breastlifts, augmentations, and reductions are commonly performed along with abdominoplasty. This combination of rejuvenation of the breast and belly yields a dramatic improvement in the overall body contour, especially following changes associated with pregnancy and childbearing. We do recommend that patients perform this when they are certain that they will not be having additional children as the results will be adversely affected by additional pregnancies.

BODY CONTOURING Similar to performing breast surgery with tummy tuck, performing body contouring including breast and fat contouring of the inner and outer thighs, hips, and/or abdomen are an excellent way to achieve better balance between the upper and lower trunk.

TEENS AND COSMETIC SURGERY

According to ASPS, the top five surgical procedures among patients 18 and younger in 2005 were:

- Breast augmentation
- Male breast reduction
- Ear surgery
- Liposuction
- Rhinoplasty

Bearing in mind that not every procedure is appropriate for every age, I advise my youngest patients and their parents to consider a few important factors:

- Wait to do your breasts until you turn 18. Some women develop later in life, and the result you see with implants may change if you grow a cup size. Gynecomastia can be performed on a boy as young as 16.

- Liposuction may seem like a quick fix to lose extra body fat, but it is still surgery. Focus on the changes you can make yourself with diet and exercise. Consider lipo a last resort.

- I am seeing many patients whose parents want to buy them a nose job for a graduation or birthday gift. Fourteen is the bare minimum at which I would recommend a nose job, as the nose fully develops in girls between 14 and 15, and in boys between 15 and 16.

- Kids can be quite cruel, and protruding ears are a stigma that can cause plenty of emotional distress through the early years. Otoplasty or pinning back the ears can be done as early as four years old.

Resources

www.greenbergcosmeticsurgery.com

www.alittlenipalittletuck.com

www.surgery.org

www.plasticsurgery.org

Index

H

Hair, 3, 7, 13, 18, 22, 90-2, 94, 98, 105-8, 122, 125-26, 132, 151-53, 157-60, 162-3, 165,169

Hair Transplant, 92

Hematoma, 24-5, 104

Hormones, 37, 65,167-8

Human Tissue Fillers, 115, 127, 143

Hyaluronic Acid, 13, 134-5, 140-2, 165

Hyaluronic Acid Gel, 140-2

Hydroquinone, 147, 169

Hylaform®, 141-2

Hyperpigmentation, 169-70

Hypertension, 81

Hypertrophic Scar, 26

I

Inamed® Silicone-Filled Breast Implants, 46

Injectables, 9, 91, 134-5, 144-5, 157

Intense Pulsed Light (IPL), 152, 155-6

Invisalign®, 172

J

Jaw, 125, 127-8, 157, 164

Jaw Implants, 128

Juvéderm™, 135-6, 141, 145

K

Keloid, 21, 26

L

Laser Hair Removal, 13, 152-3, 157-60, 165

Laser Skin Resurfacing, 145-8, 152-6, 159-60, 166

Laser Therapy, 153

Lasers, 134, 148, 152-5, 158-60

LED, 157

Lidocaine, 59, 62-3, 143

Lidocaine Toxicity, 62

Light Peels, 146

Light Sources, 152-3, 155-60, 165-6

Lip Augmentation, 164, 175

Lip Enhancement, 145

Notes